# CONTRIBUTORS

Mir H. Ali, MD, PhD
Resident
Orthopaedic Surgery
Mayo Clinic
Rochester, Minnesota

Keith R. Berend, MD
Clinical Assistant Professor
Department of Orthopaedics
The Ohio State University
Columbus, Ohio

Gurdeep S. Biring, MSc, FRCS
United Kingdom

Jeffrey L. Bush, MD
Central Maine Orthopaedics
Auburn, Maine

Clive P. Duncan, MD, MSc, FRCSC
Professor, Department of Orthopaedics,
University of British Columbia
Head, Department of Orthopaedics
Vancouver Acute Health Services
Vancouver, BC, Canada

Donald S. Garbuz, MD, FRCSC
Assistant Professor
Orthopaedics
University of British Columbia
Vancouver, BC, Canada

Kenneth Gustke, MD
Florida Orthopaedic Institute
Tampa, Florida

Stefan Kreuzer, MD, MS
Chief of Orthopaedics
Memorial Bone and Joint Clinic
Memorial Herman Memorial City Hospital
Houston, Texas

Adolph V. Lombardi Jr, MD, FACS
Clinical Assistant Professor
Department of Orthopaedics and
Department of Biomechanical Engineering
The Ohio State University
Columbus, Ohio

Joel M. Matta, MD
Director, Hip and Pelvis Institute
Saint John's Health Center
Santa Monica, California

Mark W. Pagnano, MD
Associate Professor of Orthopaedic Surgery
Mayo College of Medicine
Mayo Clinic
Rochester, Minnesota

Thomas Parker Vail, MD
Professor and Chairman
Department of Orthopaedic Surgery
University of California, San Francisco
San Francisco, California

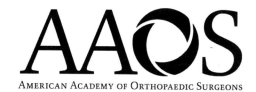

AMERICAN ACADEMY OF ORTHOPAEDIC SURGEONS

Limited Incisions for Total Hip Arthroplasty

*Published by the*
**American Academy of Orthopaedic Surgeons**
6300 North River Road
Rosemont, IL 60018
1-800-626-6726

The material presented in *Limited Incisions for Total Hip Arthroplasty* has been made available by the American Academy of Orthopaedic Surgeons for educational purposes only. This material is not intended to present the only, or necessarily best, methods or procedures for the medical situations discussed, but rather is intended to represent an approach, view, statement, or opinion of the author(s) or producer(s), which may be helpful to others who face similar situations.

Some drugs or medical devices demonstrated in Academy courses or described in Academy print or electronic publications have not been cleared by the Food and Drug Administration (FDA) or have been cleared for specific uses only. The FDA has stated that it is the responsibility of the physician to determine the FDA clearance status of each drug or device he or she wishes to use in clinical practice.

Furthermore, any statements about commercial products are solely the opinion(s) of the author(s) and do not represent an Academy endorsement or evaluation of these products. These statements may not be used in advertising or for any commercial purpose.

First Edition
Copyright © 2007 by the
American Academy of Orthopaedic Surgeons

ISBN 10: 0-89203-424-6
ISBN 13: 978-0-89203-424-6

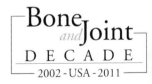

# CONTENTS

# PREFACE

Total hip arthroplasty is a wonderful operation. For the patient with disabling hip pathology, it restores function, dramatically relieves pain, and improves quality of life. It is a very gratifying operation for both the patient and the surgeon. Beginning with Sir John Charnley, surgeons have continously strived to make the procedure more durable, functional, and safer.

A recent development in this evolution has been in the actual surgical approach to the arthroplasty. Surgery performed via smaller incisions was introduced to facilitate rapid postoperative recovery. Media attention was quick and intense. Patients became increasingly knowledgeable regarding "minimally invasive surgery" and orthopaedic surgeons responded by learning these modified approaches. This monograph highlights the most frequently used current "less invasive" surgical approaches for total hip arthroplasty. The editor agrees with Clive P. Duncan, MD (Duncan CP, Toms A, Masri BA: Minimally invasive or limited incision hip replacement: Clarification and classification. *Instruc Course Lect* 2006;55:195-197.) that the term "Limited Incision Total Hip Arthoplasty" is preferable and more accurately reflects the reality of the procedure.

Five limited incision surgical approaches are presented in this monograph. The first three focus on use of an anterior approach for all or part of the procedure; the fourth approach focuses on gaining access to the joint laterally through the abductors, and the final approach is a posterior one. For ease of reference, the table of contents provides clarifications regarding the approach described in each chapter. Information on the number of incisions, approach to the hip joint, method of deep dissection, and use of fluoroscopy are included in line with the classification scheme proposed by Duncan and associates. The final chapter focuses on issues related to rapid recovery following hip replacement.

In closing, I would like to express my appreciation to the authors for their outstanding contributions and to the American Academy of Orthopaedic Surgeons for their support of this publication. It has been my pleasure to work with such talented surgeons who are leaders in this field. This monograph will prove an excellent reference for limited incision hip arthroplasty.

Mary I. O'Connor, MD
Chair, Department of Orthopaedic Surgery
Mayo Clinic
Jacksonville, Florida

# SINGLE-INCISION ANTERIOR APPROACH FOR TOTAL HIP ARTHROPLASTY: SMITH-PETERSEN APPROACH

STEFAN KREUZER, MD, MS
JOEL M. MATTA, MD

Hip replacement surgery has become one of the most successful interventions in modern medicine. The clinical results frequently show well over 90% good or excellent outcomes.[1,2] Recently, an increased emphasis has been paid to surgical approaches that lessen trauma to soft tissue and bone, potentially allowing a much quicker recovery. This has resulted in several modifications of existing techniques as well as the establishment of new techniques. Modification of the posterior and anterolateral approaches has resulted in decreased incision length and less detachment of the muscles from bone; however, the general principal of these approaches has stayed the same. The main advantages of these techniques are the familiarity to surgeons and the possibility of extensile exposure when needed. Two-incision techniques were developed with the intention of allowing each component to be placed in an optimal position with the least amount of soft-tissue damage. These approaches usually require intraoperative radiography since direct visualization of the femur often is not possible and visualization of the acetabulum may be suboptimal.

Total hip arthroplasty (THA) through a single-incision anterior approach is a less invasive technique because it does not adversely affect any of the major muscle groups around the hip joint, consisting of the hip extensors, abductors, and short external rotators.[3] Hip extensors are vital to activities of daily living such as getting out of a chair, walking upstairs, getting in and out of a car, and rising from the toilet. The abductors are critical for proper gait. The short external rotators are dynamic stabilizers of the hip joint; therefore, they are important to hip stability. Although the hip flexors are also important, they are rarely sufficiently affected during surgery to hinder hip function.

The first hip arthroplasty performed through a single anterior incision was by Robert Judet in 1947 at Hospital Raymond Poincare in Garches outside of Paris, France. The patient was supine on the Judet table that was designed by Judet's father, Henri Judet in 1940.[4,5] Judet referred to the surgical approach as the "Heuter approach." A published reference for this, however, is unknown, and "Heuter" may have been a reference to "Heuter Volkmann," the approach for drainage of a tubercular hip abscess. The approach also can be called the "Short Smith-Pete" because it follows the Smith-Petersen interval distal and lateral to the anterior superior iliac spine. Judet used the anterior approach for several reasons: (1) the hip is an anterior joint, closer to the skin anterior than posterior; (2) the approach follows an internervous plane between the superior and inferior gluteal nerves lateral (tensor fascia lata) and the femoral nerve medial (sartorius); and (3) the approach exposes the hip with minimal detachment of the muscular attachments.

This anterior approach preserves posterior structures that are important for preventing dislocation while preserving abductor muscle attachments to the greater

**FIGURE 1**

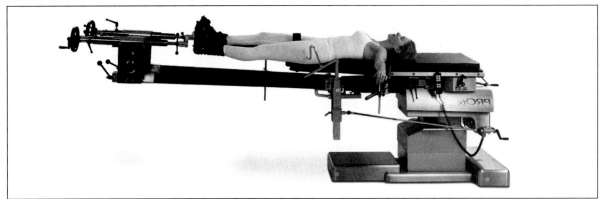

There are multiple choices that assist in holding the leg in the desired position. Shown is the PROfx table by OSI designed by JM Matta, MD, www.osiosi.com.

trochanter.[6,7] The gluteus maximum and tensor fascia lata muscles also remain undisturbed and function as hip abductors and pelvic stabilizers, inserting on the fascia lata/iliotibial band complex to form the "deltoid of the hip." Preservation of this "hip deltoid" and the attachments of the gluteus minimus and medius facilitate earlier functional recovery and avoid postoperative abduction weakness.[8,9]

Acetabular access is easy to appreciate through the anterior approach; however, femoral access is more difficult. This has lead to other techniques that often require a separate incision for implantation of the femoral stem.[10] With the single anterior incision, access to both the acetabulum and femur is facilitated by a special orthopaedic table or table attachment used to control leg positioning during the procedure.[11-14] The original table used in France by Judet was the Judet/Tasserit table. This table is no longer manufactured, which led to the design of the OSI PROfx table (**Figure 1**). We currently use the OSI PROfx and HANA (OSI, Union City, CA) tables, and the tables have the additional feature of the femoral jack and hook device to facilitate femoral exposure. Other devices, such as the arch table extension and the medacta table extension, are available. One of the authors has some experience with the arch table extension; the other devices are only included for the sake of completeness. In this chapter, we will review patient selection criteria, surgical technique, pearls and pitfalls, and early to midterm clinic results of the single-incision anterior approach using a special operating table.

## PATIENT SELECTION

Although the single-incision anterior approach with a specialized surgical table for hip replacement can be performed in most patients, certain patients are not considered appropriate candidates for this approach. Patients with severe heterotopic bone, ipsilateral below-knee amputation, an ipsilateral hinged knee prosthesis, or severe dysplasia requiring femoral osteotomy should undergo hip arthroplasty via a different surgical approach. In severe heterotopic bone, femoral exposure and mobilization may be very difficult. In below-knee amputation, a proximal tibial pin may be attached to a Kirschner traction bow that attaches to the table spar, but this adds complexity to the procedure. Although ipsilateral total knee arthroplasty is not an absolute contraindication, a hinged knee may rotate out around the rotating platform. Caution should be used since we do not have any experience with this particular situation. Although acetabular dysplasia in need of bone grafting can be done without difficulty by fixing the graft with either screws or a plate, a femoral shortening osteotomy can be difficult. Acetabular work (ie, bone graft with screw fixation) is relatively easy, but the difficulty with dysplastic hips is on the femoral side. Dyplastic hips that require femoral shortening osteotomy are difficult to correct and require a separate incision. Therefore, we feel that dysplasia with the need for femoral shortening osteotomy is a contraindication. Femoral dysplasia without femoral shortening is acceptable. The advantage of using the anterior approach in dysplasia includes preservation of the musculature, radiographic control of reaming that allows the surgeon to more accurately and confidently medialize the reamer, and the ability to confirm being in the true rather than a false acetabulum. Previous radiation to the hip region also may cause difficulty with exposure and femoral mobilization. Although some surgeons promote the anterior approach for hip revisions (K Keggi, MD, personal communication, 2004), it is more difficult because of the inability of extensile exposure of the femur and not having direct visual access of the intramedullary canal. Acetabular exposure actually may be easier since the Smith-Petersen approach is the only true extensile approach to the hip because it follows the only true internervous and intermuscular plane. We actually prefer the anterior approach particularly for some difficult acetabular problems and acetabular revisions when the femoral component will be left undisturbed. Polyethylene liner exchanges can be done through the anterior approach with little or no difficulty.

Factors that make the anterior approach more difficult are: (1) increased body mass index (BMI), especially in men (**Figure 2**), (2) large, muscular men, (3) patients with large trochanters that have a "hook" medial to the intramedullary canal (**Figure 3**), and (4) hips with very small offset and a broad iliac wing. Severe osteopenia can increase the risk of intraoperative fracture at the calcar or the ankle. The ideal patient is a woman with reasonable offset and BMI and with good bone quality. Hemiarthroplasty also can be performed, but placement of the unipolar or bipolar head sometimes may be difficult because of soft-tissue constraints. Manipulating the leg spar may be of great assistance.

## PREOPERATIVE PATIENT EDUCATION

As with all surgical procedures, preoperative patient education is paramount. Routine surgical complications should be discussed as it relates to hip arthroplasty and devices used. Additional points should be discussed as they appear to be unique to the anterior approach, including an increased incidence of lateral thigh numbness that usually resolves within a few months, an occasional seroma requiring aspiration, and a higher incidence of trochanteric bursitis if femoral offset is increased over normal because the iliotibial band is not "released" with the anterior approach. The numbness is

**FIGURE 2**

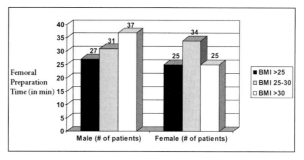

Graph showing an apparent close correlation between surgical time and BMI in men but not in women.

most likely caused by the stretching or cutting of a small superficial branch exiting laterally off the lateral femoral cutaneous nerve (**Figure 4**). Most patients are very accepting of the slight decrease in feeling over the lateral thigh, especially if they have been properly educated prior to surgery. Lateral cutaneous nerve palsy does not appear to occur with proper placement of the skin incision and with avoidance of aggressive medial retraction of soft tissue. Postoperative seroma is easily treated with aspiration and a spica dressing. It usually occurs in thin female patients and rarely requires more than one aspiration. Trochanteric bursitis occurs more commonly and is easily treated with a steroid injection and physical therapy. Preoperative education is important to reduce patient anxiety should these problems occur. For surgeons unfamiliar with this approach, potential complications related to the learning curve may need to be discussed. If the anterior capsule is repaired, the patient is instructed to avoid external rotation in hyperextension for 6 weeks. We also review with patients the "extreme" posterior precautions that include the combination of hyperflexion, adduction, and more than 45° of internal rotation.

## SURGICAL TECHNIQUE

Although the single-incision anterior approach can be performed without a special surgical table, our main experience is with the use of a specialty surgical table. We also believe that the technique is significantly facilitated by the use of a specialty table (**Figure 1**) or the use of special devices to position the extremity (**Figure 5**). Dis-

**FIGURE 3**

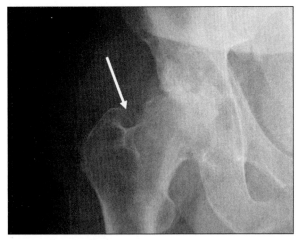

Radiograph showing a large trochanter with a significant hook that resulted in a more difficult femoral exposure.

**FIGURE 4**

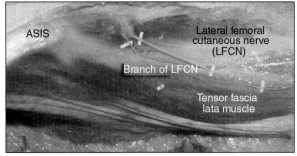

The lateral femoral cutaneous nerve has a small branch that results in peri-incisional numbness that usually resolves with time.

cussion of the surgical technique will be limited to the technique that we perform on the OSI PROfx table.

## Patient Positioning

After preoperative templating of radiographs, the patient is placed in the supine position on an orthopaedic table. The operative leg is placed into a leg-holding device that allows controlled positioning of the leg in space during surgery. The leg is not draped free but is attached to the leg spar to allow traction, rotation, extension, and adduction (**Figure 1**). The contralateral hip is placed in neutral rotation, extension, and abduction-adduction to serve as a radiographic control for the operated side. The operative leg is set in slight internal rotation to enhance the landmark of the natural bulge of the tensor fascia lata muscle. Pneumatic compression boots can be applied to both legs for intraoperative deep venous thrombosis (DVT) prophylaxis.

## Exposure

The incision is placed 2 cm posterior and 2 cm distal to the anterior superior iliac spine (ASIS). This straight incision is extended in a distal and slightly posterior direction to a point 2 to 3 cm anterior to the greater trochanter (**Figure 6**), for a total of 6 to 10 cm. The sub-

cutaneous tissue is undermined to allow the placement of the retractor or protractor for the protection of the skin and to avoid maceration of the skin edges. The aponeurosis of the tensor fascia lata is incised in line with the skin incision and the direction of the muscle fibers. The interval between the tensor and sartorius is developed by blunt dissection with the index finger around the medial aspect of the tensor within the sheath of the incised aponeurosis. Continued blunt dissection along the medial tensor in the posterior and proximal directions allows palpation of the lateral hip capsule. A cobra retractor is placed along the superolateral hip capsule. A Hibbs retractor is used to retract the sartorius and rectus femoris medially, exposing the reflected head of the rectus. More distally in the wound, electro bovie cautery is used to incise the fascia over the rectus femoris to isolate the lateral femoral circumflex vessels which are then tied with a free tie or carefully coagulated. These vessels can bleed briskly and attention to detail avoids extensive blood loss (**Figure 7**). The precapsular fat is then identified and excised for adequate visualization of the capsule. Again, adequate coagulation of precapsular vessels is necessary to avoid excessive bleeding. The reflected head of the rectus and the iliocapsularis muscles are gently lifted off the capsule and a second cobra retractor is then placed on the medial hip capsule (**Figure 8**). Alternatively, a Hibbs retractor can be used to avoid retraction of the rectus and iliocapsularis until after the arthrotomy is done. Additional distal splitting of the aponeurosis that overlies the anterior capsule enhances the exposure of the origin of the vastus lateralis muscle.

**FIGURE 5**

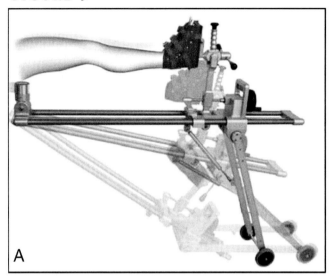
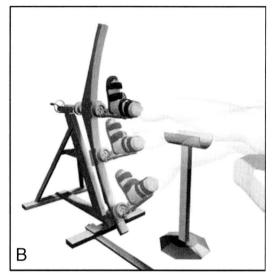

Examples of devices that assist in holding the leg in the desired position. **A,** Medacta table extension. **B,** Arch table extension.

**FIGURE 6**

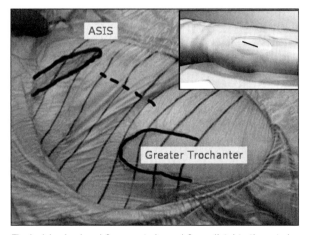

The incision is placed 2 cm posterior and 2 cm distal to the anterior superior iliac spine (ASIS). This straight incision is extended in a distal and slightly posterior direction to a point 2 to 3 cm anterior to the greater trochanter for a total of 6 to 10 cm.

**FIGURE 7**

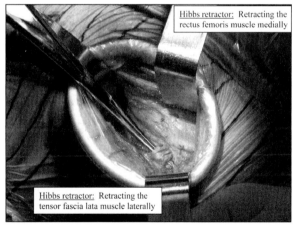

The lateral femoral circumflex vessels are ligated with free tie or carefully coagulated. These vessels can bleed briskly, and attention to detail avoids extensive blood loss during the surgery.

The capsulotomy is done in an L-shaped or upside down T-shaped fashion (**Figure 9**). The distal portion of the lateral capsule is detached from the sulcus between the anterolateral neck and greater trochanter and from the superior acetabular rim next to the insertion of the reflected head of the rectus. The distal portion of the medial flap of the capsule is detached from the femur at the anterior intertrochanteric line down to the lesser trochanter. Frequently there is brisk bleeding from the cut edges of the capsule. The medial and lateral flaps are

FIGURE 8

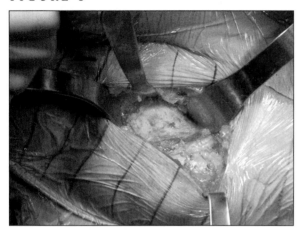

The reflected head of the rectus and the iliocapsularis muscles are lifted off the capsule and two cobra retractors are placed to expose the capsule.

FIGURE 9

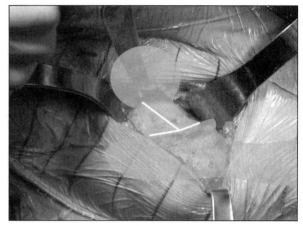

The capsulotomy is done in an L-shaped or T-shaped fashion. Tag suture can be placed in each flap to facilitate manipulation of the capsule during reaming.

tagged to assist with retraction, especially during acetabular reaming and for subsequent repair. The cobra retractors are now replaced inside the capsule, exposing the femoral neck.

## Hip Dislocation

Preliminary hip dislocation before the neck osteotomy is not essential; however, it can greatly facilitate exposure of the posterior and medial neck and improve mobilization of the femur for subsequent preparation. Infrequently, dislocation may be difficult because of protrusio or previous acetabular fracture, or massive acetabular osteophytes. In these unusual cases, the neck is cut in situ. To dislocate the hip, a narrow Hohmann retractor is placed on the anterolateral acetabular rim to allow excision of the anterolateral labrum, anterolateral osteophytes, and/or ossified labrum with an osteotome, thereby exposing the articulation. Distal traction on the extremity creates a small gap between the femoral head and the roof of the acetabulum. A femoral head skid (Aesculap, Central Valley, PA) can be placed into the gap. By sliding it medially, the ligamentum teres can then be released, thereby freeing up the femoral head of all attachments. The traction is then partially released, and external rotation of the limb allows the hip to be dislocated anteriorly. External rotation of the femur is accomplished by rotation of the leg spar rotation wheel. If the patient is very osteoporotic, undue force from the rotation wheel can fracture the tibia or ankle. For this reason, two modifications were incorporated to aid in the dislocation procedure. The scrubbed surgical assistant can aid dislocation by grasping the femoral condyles and applying additional rotation, therefore decreasing the torque applied to the distal extremity. Preferentially, a femoral head corkscrew can be placed into the head before dislocation and can be used to pull and externally rotate the femoral head. By combining the corkscrew and skid and unlocking the table rotation control, the head can be dislocated without applying any distal rotational force to the extremity. After dislocation, the hip is externally rotated 90°. A narrow Hohmann retractor is placed distal to the lesser trochanter and beneath the vastus lateralis origin. The medial capsular flap is retracted medialward to expose the hip capsule which remains attached to the medial and posterior femoral neck. This capsule is then released, exposing the lesser trochanter down the posterior aspect of the femoral neck. The hip is reduced back into the acetabulum by internal rotation, and the neck cut is completed in situ. This dislocation procedure should be fairly easy if adequate capsule is released initially. If the surgeon feels that excessive torque is required to dislocate the hip, an in situ neck osteotomy should be done.

## Neck Osteotomy and Extraction of the Femoral Head

With the cobra retractors placed around the medial and lateral neck, a reciprocating saw can be used to safely osteotomize the femoral neck at the templated level (**Figure 10**). The neck cut is completed with an osteotome that divides the lateral neck from the medial greater trochanter, and should be directed posterior and slightly medial to avoid fracture of the greater trochanter. The femoral head corkscrew is used to remove the head with care, protecting the tensor from laceration by the sharp edge of the neck as it is extracted. Alternatively, a double osteotomy may be done by adding a second osteotomy approximately at the level of the articular cartilage border of the femoral head. With the assistance of a threaded Steinmann pin, the wedge and the head are easily removed. Care must be taken not to plunge with the saw blade because this can result in a cut into the posterior wall of the acetabulum. If extensive bleeding at the osteotomy site is encountered, bone wax can be placed on the osteotomy site.

## Acetabular Preparation

Preparation of the acetabulum is facilitated by careful placement of retractors, removal of the labrum and osteophytes, and careful guidance with the image intensifier. External rotation of the femur to about 45° facilitates acetabular exposure. Light traction also limits femoral interference. Too much traction tightens the iliopsoas and pulls the femur into an anterior obstructing position. A bent Hohmann retractor is placed over the anterior rim of the acetabulum to retract the anterior muscle; care should be taken to avoid perforation of the anterior musculature and soft tissues. A cobra retractor is placed posteriorly with the tip on the mid-posterior rim (**Figure 11**). The labrum should be carefully excised, and the prominent band of the inferior capsule incised longitudinally perpendicular to the band to facilitate placement of the acetabular liner. Acetabular reaming can then be done with fluoroscopic guidance (**Figure 11**). After each reamer, finger palpation helps to ensure avoidance of reaming too anteriorly or posteriorly. If the neck cut is left too long, it can interfere with the insertion of the acetabular reamer. A re-cut of the neck should then be done.

## Acetabular Cup Insertion

Acetabular cup insertion is facilitated with a curved or offset handle inserter that reduces pressure on the distal wound and avoids placing the component too vertical. The tendency with this technique is to place the cup in a too anteverted and vertical position because of the soft-tissue interference with the cup inserter. To ensure accuracy of component position, image intensification can be used to verify the abduction angle and anteversion as the prosthesis is sequentially seated (**Figure 11**). Anteversion can be difficult to judge if the patient is not positioned carefully on the operative table. Finger palpation of the native acetabular rim can be a secondary check for accurate acetabular cup placement. The appropriate liner is then inserted and any overhanging acetabular osteophytes are removed with a curved ½-inch osteotome.

## Femoral Exposure

Femoral exposure is the most challenging step and is aided by the leg-holding device and a femoral hook. The hook attaches to a hook bracket which is attached to the operating table. It is designed to facilitate exposure of the femur through the small anterior incision. After acetabular insertion, the gross traction control on the leg is used to release all the traction and the femur is internally rotated to neutral. The femoral hook is placed just distal to the vastus ridge and around the posterior femur. The femur is externally rotated 90°, hyperextended, and adducted with the assistance of the leg-holding device. This maneuver should be slow and deliberate to ensure that the greater trochanter is not caught behind the posterior acetabular wall. The hook is then attached to the most convenient hole on the bracket, which is attached to a jack on the table. Elevation of the jack causes the hook to deliver the proximal femur anteriorly, aiding femoral preparation. Sequential releases of the posterior capsule are essential and will facilitate femoral mobilization.

Five sequential releases allow reproducible femoral exposure and are as follows: (1) Superior capsular: the superior capsular release is done from the superior acetabulum rim in a subperiosteal fashion. The initial inverted T incision can be converted into an H-type incision to improve femoral exposure. (2) Inferior capsular: capsule is released from the inferior neck along the

FIGURE 10

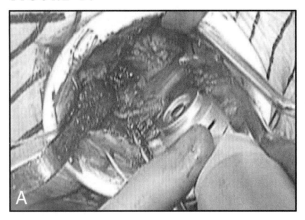 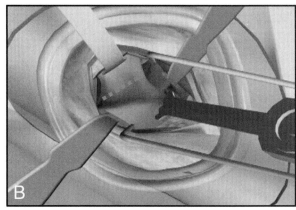

With the cobra retractors placed around the medial and lateral neck, a reciprocating saw can be used to safely osteotomize the femoral neck at the templated level. **A,** Oscillating saw cutting the femoral neck. **B,** Dotted line indicates the osteotomy site.

FIGURE 11

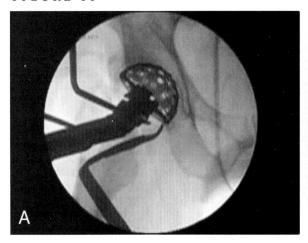 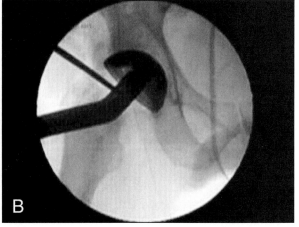

To ensure accuracy of component position, image intensification can be used to verify the abduction angle and anteversion during reaming and placement of the acetabular component. **A,** Radiographic visualization during reaming. **B,** Radiographic visualization during acetabular cup insertion.

intertrochanteric line, if not done during the dislocation step or as described earlier. Bleeding can be encountered. (3) Piriformis recess: further releases may be necessary along the piriformis recess. (4) Posterior capsular: capsule can be released along the posterior neck of the femur. The tip of the greater trochanter can then be delivered through the posterior lateral capsule release and past the posterior wall of the acetabulum. As the femur is elevated, the surgeon should monitor the tension on the leg during elevation of the hook because too

much tension may cause fracture of the trochanter. (5) Short external rotators: rarely, the short external rotators need to be released along the piriformis recess and the posterior femur.

A cobra or Ranawat retractor is placed with its tip on the posterior femoral neck, and a trochanteric retractor (bent Hohmann or 90° Hohmann) is placed over the tip of the trochanter. The lateral capsular flap may need to be detached from the base of the neck in an anterior to posterior direction, further facilitating exposure of the medial greater trochanter and enhancing femoral mobility. Any lateral neck remnant is excised with a rongeur.

## Femoral Broaching

Although any stem can be used with this approach, stems requiring straight reamers for canal preparation are more difficult because they require more mobilization of the femur to allow access down the canal. We prefer systems that offer an offset broach handle, which are easily introduced into the proximal femur without further release of the soft tissues. If further mobilization of the femur is necessary, it can be accomplished with additional release of the capsule and infrequently with sequential releases of the obturator internus and piriformis tendons. Further mobilization of the femur should not be accomplished with further elevation of the hook past a point of excessive tension on the leg because this can lead to fracture of the greater trochanter. Slight Trendelenburg can also assist to gain additional clearance for the broach handle. The obturator internus tendon inserts inside the internal lip of the posterior aspect of the greater trochanter, and in difficult cases it may be released to allow additional immobilization of the femur. Likewise, release of the piriformis may be done in extreme cases. The release of these rotators is preferred over the release of the obturator externus, which exerts a more medial pull and which we consider to be most important in hip stability.

Broaching is accomplished with the tip of the broach entering the neck near the posterior medial cortex (**Figure 12**). Care must be taken to ensure that the broach is not in excessive anteversion, which may occur if the femur is not externally rotated enough. It is possible to perforate the posterior or lateral femoral cortex because of the interference of the patient's soft tissues on the broach handle (**Figure 13**). Broaching is continued to an appropriate size based on intraoperative feel, insertion length, and preoperative templating. The appropriate trial neck and head are placed onto the broach as determined by the preoperative templating, and by its observed relationship to the tip of the greater trochanter. After the hook is lowered and removed, a trial reduction is done to confirm proper limb lengthening and hip stability. The hip is easily reduced with internal rotation and slight traction.

## Final Review: Hip Stability and Closure

The limb length and offset determination can be confirmed with an intraoperative AP pelvis radiograph or with the use of an image intensifier (**Figure 14**). An image of the contralateral hip should be obtained and printed, and then placed on the screen. The operated hip is imaged, and the rotation, abduction, and flexion are adjusted to position the hip equivalent with the contralateral side. The image is printed, and the two images are compared by superimposing the transparencies. The bony landmarks of the femurs are aligned, and the pelvic landmarks compared. With the trial components inserted, anterior hip stability is checked in extension and external rotation by applying rotation to the leg to 85° of external rotation. Posterior stability also can be tested by removing the boot from the leg spar, flexing the hip to 90°, internally rotating to 45°, and adducting to 20° (**Figure 15**). If the hip dislocates during manipulation, it is necessary to check for acetabular osteophytes that may cause impingement. Once the trial components are chosen, the hook is replaced around the posterior femur, traction is applied, and the hip is dislocated with slight traction and external rotation. The femur is repositioned into the preparation position (90°+ external rotation, hyperextension, adduction, and hook elevation). The trial components are removed and the final components are inserted. The image intensifier is used to confirm position of the acetabulum and correctness of limb length and offset. Inevitably there may be some variability of soft-tissue tension between individuals, and with the anterior approach it does not appear to be necessary to create an abnormal increased offset or increased limb length to tension the soft tissues.

The wound is checked for bleeding and the anterior and lateral capsular tag sutures are tied together. Additional capsular closure may be done if desired. The fascia lata is closed with a running suture, followed by subcutaneous and skin closure. We place both deep and superficial drains.

## PITFALLS TO AVOID IN SURGICAL TECHNIQUE/COMMON ERRORS

This section covers common pitfalls, how to avoid complications, and how to deal with complications when they occur.

**FIGURE 12**

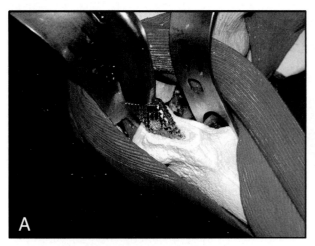
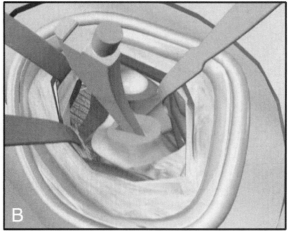

Broaching is accomplished with the tip of the broach entering the neck near the posterior medial cortex. A broach-only system with an offset broach handle facilitates the preparation of the femur. **A,** Offset broach handle to facilitate entering the femoral canal. **B,** Insertion of the final implant.

## Dislocation and Limb-length Inequality

The incidence of dislocation using the anterior one-incision approach is very low because of the preservation of dynamic hip stabilizer (short external rotators). Nevertheless, prevention by proper placement of components and intraoperative stability testing is important. An intraoperative radiograph will not only confirm proper placement of components for hip stability, but it also gives valuable information about offset and limb length. Because of the increased stability of the anterior approach, leg lengthening to gain stability is rarely necessary.[12] Because the patient is in the supine position, a high quality radiograph can be obtained.

## Intraoperative Crack, Periprosthetic Fracture, and Lateral Perforation

### Intraoperative Calcar Crack
An intraoperative calcar crack of the proximal femur can occur with aggressive broaching. Although we find that cerclage wires can be passed around the proximal femur without extending the 10-cm incision, the approach can be extended distally and laterally, elevating the vastus to expose more of the femur as needed. A small crack can be treated with one cerclage wire above

the lesser trochanter. Extension past the lesser trochanter may require a second wire (**Figure 16**). Manipulating the leg in the reduced position with the leg-holding device greatly facilitates the passage of the cerclage wire/cable.

### Periprosthetic Fracture
An acute postoperative fracture is somewhat more challenging but also can be treated without much additional exposure. If noted intraoperatively, an additional separate lateral incision over the vastus lateralis can be made and two additional wires can be passed. The implant should be removed prior to placement of the wire and reinserted once confirmation of anatomic reduction of the fracture is confirmed. The same approach can be used if the fracture is noted in the first few weeks. Conversion to a more fully coated straight stem that can be inserted via the anterior approach is possible, but it will require slightly more releases around the femur (**Figure 16**). If no perforation occurred during surgery, four cerclage wires should be sufficient. The postoperative course should be modified to touch-down weight bearing for at least 6 weeks.

### Lateral Perforation
If lateral perforation occurs during broaching (**Figure 17**), it must be noted early to avoid broaching up and

**FIGURE 13**

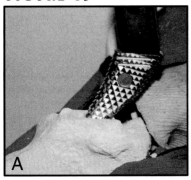
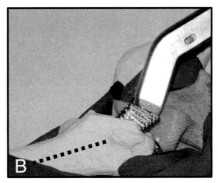
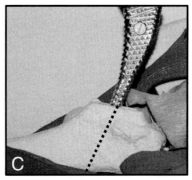

**A,** Correct direction of insertion of broach handle to avoid perforation. **B,** Fully inserted broach. Dashed line shows correct direction of insertion. **C,** Incorrect direction of insertion of broach with risk of lateral perforation. Dashed line shows incorrect direction.

**FIGURE 14**

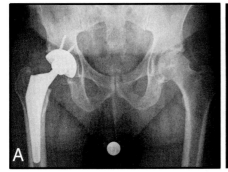
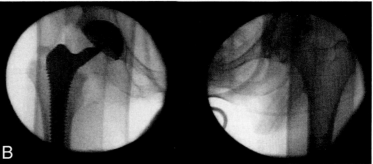

The leg length and offset determination can be confirmed with an intraoperative AP pelvis radiograph **(A)** or with the use of an image intensifier **(B)**. The image is printed, and the two images are compared by superimposing the transparencies.

**FIGURE 15**

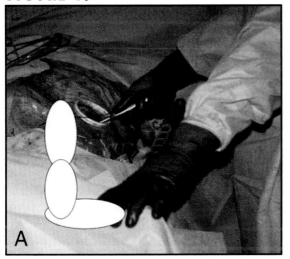
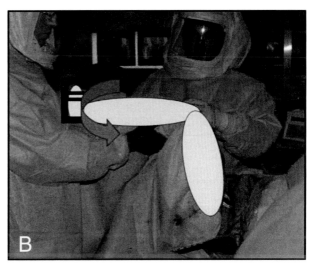

With the trial components inserted, **(A)** anterior hip stability is checked in extension and external rotation by applying rotation to the leg to 85° of external rotation. **B,** Posterior stability can be tested by removing the boot from the leg-holding device, flexing the hip to 90°, internally rotating to 45°, and adducting to 20°.

**FIGURE 16**

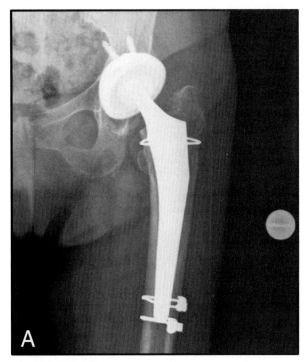
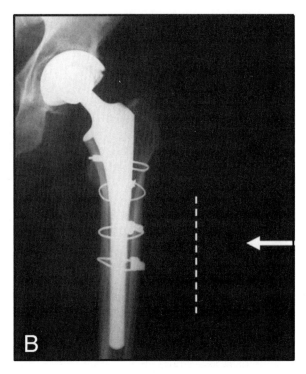

Radiographs representing two separate patients that required additional fixation for intraoperative fractures. **A,** Radiograph showing an intraoperative fracture that was noted to have extended distally. The treatment included removal of the stem with placement of three cerclage wires. Although the stem had slight subsidence initially, it went on to stable fixation and an excellent result. **B,** The patient sustained a fall in the hospital on the second postoperative day and was noted to have a fracture that propagated distally. The patient required a return to the OR to remove the original stem, followed by stabilization of the fracture with four cerclage wires and reimplantation with a longer revision-type stem.

increasing the size of the perforation. If a lateral perforation is suspected, the image intensifier can be used for confirmation. The postoperative regimen may be modified to touch-down weight bearing, but no other treatment is necessary. An intraoperative radiograph should be obtained to ensure that no other fractures occurred.

## Unstable Acetabular Component

Due to the unfamiliarity with this approach, in the early learning curve occasionally it may be difficult to obtain a stable cup. This may result from excessive reaming anteriorly or posteriorly. It is advisable to intermittently palpate the anterior and posterior wall with the index finger between reamers to ensure concentric reaming. If the cup appears to be unstable, downsize the reamer and medialize the reamer to the teardrop. If difficulty continues, a suboptimal version may gain cup stability by increasing acetabular cup coverage. Multiple screws also may be necessary for supplemental fixation. In this case, a lipped or face-changing liner may be needed to obtain a stable hip joint. A slight compensation in version during femoral broaching may also avoid future instability.

## POSTOPERATIVE CARE INCLUDING PHYSICAL THERAPY AND PAIN MANAGEMENT PROTOCOLS

Provided that the patient has adequate bone quality, weight bearing as tolerated is allowed after surgery with minimal postoperative restrictions. Walking with the aid of a crutch, cane, or walker is based on individual patient

**FIGURE 17**

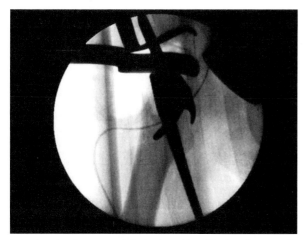

Lateral perforation occurred during broaching. The broach was redirected and the patient was kept on touch-down weight bearing for 4 to 6 weeks.

ability. Gait training and stair ambulation during the patient's hospital stay is monitored and instructed by physical therapists. Drains are discontinued on the first or second postoperative day. Most patients are discharged on postoperative day 2 or 3. Transfer to skilled nursing is rarely necessary unless there are social issues. Outpatient physical therapy is only ordered if requested by the patient or if the patient's progress in the hospital is slow. Follow-up visits include first 2 weeks postoperative, 6 weeks postoperative (only if patient has difficulty at the 2-week visit), 3 months or 6 months, and annually thereafter. Dr. Matta's protocol is 6 weeks, 1 year, and then at 2-year intervals after surgery.

Pain protocol includes regional anesthesia whenever possible and an intraoperative injection of ketorolac tromethamine (30 mg), ropivacaine (2 mg/kg), morphine (5 mg), and epinephrine (0.6 mL [1:1,000]) after closure through the drain tube. Drain suction is avoided for the first 4 hours postoperatively. It is important to note that we have observed two cases (out of 410 cases) of a 12-hour temporary foot drop postoperatively, most likely due to this cocktail of local anesthetic affecting the sciatic nerve. We do not directly inject into the capsule or musculature around the hip joint. Patients will receive a morphine PCA but are encouraged to start using oral pain medication as soon as possible. They are sent home with a prescription of narcotics. Patients also receive

indomethacin for 10 days to avoid the formation of heterotopic bone formation. Dr. Matta's protocol does not include wound injections, although morphine may be used with the spinal. Postoperatively, the patient typically receives only oral narcotics and is not prescribed the use of a PCA or indomethacin.

## CLINICAL RESULTS AND COMPLICATIONS

Dr. Matta's series of 437 consecutive, unselected patients who had 494 primary total hip arthroplasty surgeries done through an anterior approach on an orthopaedic table from September 1996 to September 2004 were reviewed. The Judet/Tasserit table was used until the PROfx table became available in January 2003 and was used subsequently. There were 54 hybrid and 442 uncemented hips in the 437 patients (57 bilateral). The average patient age was 64 years. Radiographic analysis showed an average abduction angle of 42°, with 96% in the range of 35° to 50° abduction. The average cup anteversion was 19°, with 93% within the target range of 10° to 25°. Postoperative limb-length discrepancy averaged 3 ± 2 mm (range, 0 to 26 mm). Three patients sustained dislocations for an overall dislocation rate of 0.61%. No patients required revision surgery for recurrent dislocations. There were 17 surgical complications, including one deep infection, three wound infections, one transient femoral nerve palsy, three greater trochanter fractures, two femoral shaft fractures, four calcar fractures, and three ankle fractures. In reference to the three ankle fractures, they occurred over a 2-month period in 2003. The fractures occurred when Dr. Matta changed his technique from cutting the neck in situ to dislocating the hip prior to cutting it. All three fractures occurred in elderly women with osteoporosis when attempting to dislocate the hip with torsion applied to the leg. Following these occurrences, the technique for dislocation was changed to the current femoral head skid, femoral head cork screw combination, and no or minimal distal leg torque. Since this change, the complication has not recurred. Surgical time averaged 75 minutes (range, 40 to 150 minutes), and the average blood loss was 350 mL (range, 100 to 1,300 mL). The mean hospital stay was 3 days (range, 1 to 17 days).

## CONCLUSION/DISCUSSION

For a new technique to be successful, it has to be safe, reproducible, applicable to most patients, and teachable. We feel that the anterior approach on the orthopaedic table is a minimally invasive technique applicable to all primary hip patients and can be reproduced safely. Careful surgical technique avoids complications and allows accurate and reproducible component positioning and limb-length restoration and does not increase the rate of hip dislocation. The use of this surgical technique even eliminates dislocation precautions. The fact that Dr. Matta's published series does not include any recurrent dislocators or need for revision for dislocation is significant. We feel that cadaver courses are necessary to properly teach this technique to surgeons unfamiliar with the Smith-Petersen approach.

As one begins a new technique, whether it is the originating surgeon or those subsequently learning the technique, there may be an increase in complications or an observance of new ones. Although we consider the observed complications to date to be acceptable and rarely a long-term problem, we do not consider the rates to be fixed. We also feel that reporting them and discussing them will lead to a long-term decrease in their incidence and a shortened learning curve for new surgeons. The response and enthusiasm of patients regarding their results has pushed us to continue our use of this technique and to work to address the technical details.

## REFERENCES

1. Caracciolo B, Giaquinto S: Determinants of the subjective functional outcome of total joint arthroplasty. *Arch Gerontol Geriatr* 2005;41:169-176.

2. Rissanen P, Aro S, Sintonen H, Slatis P, Paavolainen P: Quality of life and functional ability in hip and knee replacements: A prospective study. *Qual Life Res* 1996;5:56-64.

3. Matta JM: Anterior approach for total hip replacement: Background and operative technique, in Scuderi GR, Tria AJ, Berger RA (eds): *MIS Techniques in Orthopaedics.* Berlin, Springer Science & Business Media Inc, 2005, pp 121-140.

4. Judet R, Judet J: Technique and results with the acrylic femoral head prosthesis. *J Bone Joint Surg Br* 1952;34:173-180.

5. Kennon RE, Keggi JM, Wetmore RS, Zatorski LE, Huo MH, Keggi KJ: Total hip arthroplasty through a minimally invasive anterior surgical approach. *J Bone Joint Surg Am* 2003;85:39-48.

6. Bourne RB, Rorabeck CH: Soft tissue balancing: The hip. *J Arthroplasty* 2002;17:17-22.

7. DeWal H, Su E, DiCesare PE: Instability following total hip arthroplasty. *Am J Orthop* 2003;32:377-382.

8. Masonis JL, Bourne RB: Surgical approach, abductor function, and total hip arthroplasty dislocation. *Clin Orthop Relat Res* 2002;405:46-53.

9. Siguier T, Siguier M, Brumpt B: Mini-incision anterior approach does not increase dislocation rate: A study of 1037 total hip replacements. *Clin Orthop Relat Res* 2004;426:164-171.

10. Berger RA: Total hip arthroplasty using the minimally invasive two-incision approach. *Clin Orthop Relat Res* 2003;417:232-241.

11. Beaule PE, Griffin DB, Matta JM: The Levine anterior approach for total hip replacement as the treatment for an acute acetabular fracture. *J Orthop Trauma* 2004;18:623-629.

12. Matta JM, Ferguson TA: The anterior approach for hip replacement. *Orthopedics* 2005;28:927-928.

13. Yerasimides JG, Matta JM: Primary total hip arthroplasty with a minimally invasive anterior approach. *Semin Arthroplasty* 2005;16:186-190.

14. Matta JM, Shahrdar C, Ferguson T: Single-incision anterior approach for total hip arthroplasty on an orthopaedic table. *Clin Orthop Relat Res* 2005;441:115-124.

# CHAPTER 2

# LIMITED INCISION HIP ARTHROPLASTY: TWO-INCISION APPROACH

MIR H. ALI, MD, PHD
MARK W. PAGNANO, MD

Two-incision less invasive (LIS) total hip arthroplasty (THA) was introduced in 2002 with widespread media coverage that generated substantial patient and surgeon interest. However, no peer-reviewed scientific data accompanied those early reports. While the initial surgeon-developer experience was strikingly positive,[1,2] subsequent clinical series and cadaver studies have yielded more modest results.[3,4] Since 2003, these reports have looked at surgeon proficiency, clinical outcomes, and complications of two-incision LIS-THA. The most revealing of these studies have compared patients undergoing two-incision LIS-THA with patients undergoing standard open THA or other methods of LIS-THA.

This chapter describes the most common technique for two-incision LIS-THA, outlines the common errors and complications, discusses the experience at our institution, and interprets the accumulated data.

## SELECTION OF PATIENTS

Different patient selection criteria have been applied by various surgeons employing two-incision LIS-THA. Over the last few years, however, it has become clear that some subgroups of patients are more difficult to treat with a two-incision approach. Those groups include elderly women with osteoporotic bone,

markedly obese patients (BMI > 35 mg/kg$^2$), heavily muscular men, and patients with substantial bony deformity (especially those with prior fracture, retained hardware, and/or residual dysplasia). While it is possible to perform the procedure in these patients, the prevalence of complications is higher.

The initial report on two-incision LIS-THA included 75 men and 25 women, with a mean age of 55 years (range: 30 to 76 years).[1] The average weight of the patients was 80 kg (176 lb), with a range of 46 to 120 kg (102 to 265 lb). Patients were excluded if they were older than age 75, morbidly obese, or had abnormal hip anatomy, prior hip surgery, or congenital hip dysplasia. The prevalence of complications in this selected group of patients was notably low.

In contrast, the series of patients undergoing the procedure at the Mayo Clinic from March 2003 to April 2004 included 45 women and 35 men, with a mean age of 70.5 years (range: 40 to 88 years).[4] The mean weight of these patients was 93 kg (range: 63.5 to 176.5 kg [140 to 388 lb]). Patients were excluded if any of the following were present: more complex deformities, including Crowe type II dysplasia, posttraumatic degenerative arthritis, and protrusio acetabular defects. This series had an older mean patient age, a larger proportion of women, and patients with greater mean weights than the patients in the other studies. Some substantial complications were encountered in this unselected series of patients.

The demographics and exclusion criteria of the large series of two-incision LIS-THAs is summarized in **Table 1**.

## PREOPERATIVE PATIENT EDUCATION

### Outpatient

Some surgeons have championed two-incision LIS-THA as an outpatient procedure. Berger and associates[5] demonstrated that patients scheduled for surgery as the first case of the surgical day had a high likeli-hood of same-day discharge. That protocol included extensive preoperative education with a nurse and physical therapist. All patients attended a class where a nurse explained the hospital course and the expecta-tion of same-day dismissal. A physical therapy session was used for gait training with crutches with patients instructed that they would ambulate the evening of surgery. The elimination of traditional precautions after THA was emphasized.

### Inpatient

At our institution, no attempt was made to perform the surgery on an outpatient basis. Prior to surgery, all

TABLE 1

**Demographic Data and Exclusion Criteria in the Large Series of Two-incision Less Invasive Total Hip Arthroplasties**

| Study | # of Patients | Male/Female (%) | Average Age (yrs) | Average Weight (kg) | Pertinent Findings |
|---|---|---|---|---|---|
| Berger (2003) | 100 | 75/25 | 55.0 | 80.0 | 17% of all THAs done by surgeon that year. Morbidly obese patients with abnormal hip anatomy or prior surgery or dislocation excluded. |
| Mears, et al (2003) | 275 | 60/40 | 59.0 | 85.0 | Multicenter trial. Patients with any major comorbidities, previous hip surgery, or osteoporosis excluded. |
| Archibeck & White (2004) | 479 | 52/48 | 61.0 | 77.6 | Industry-sponsored. 159 different surgeons. Average BMI = 26 kg/m². |
| Pagnano, et al (2005) | 80 | 44/56 | 70.5 | 93.0 | Patients with complex deformities, posttraumatic arthritis, and protrusion acetabular defects excluded. |
| Bal, et al (2005) | 89 | 64/36 | 58.5 | 91.5 | Patients with history of surgery on ipsilateral hip and/or preexisting hip deformity excluded. BMI = 30.7 kg/m². |

patients attended an optional seminar on total hip and total knee arthroplasty at the Mayo Clinic. These seminars explained the upcoming patient hospitalization, aspects of postoperative physical therapy, pain control, and long-term lifestyle adjustments required by a patient with a total joint replacement. The patients were also counseled on discharge options and criteria. All patients were encouraged to proceed with weight bearing as tolerated and to eliminate all ambulatory aides as soon as comfortable.

## SURGICAL TECHNIQUE

The most commonly used two-incision surgical approach is the technique described by Mears and Berger[1,2,6] (two-incision LIS-THA with intraoperative fluoroscopy). The patient is prepped and draped in the usual sterile fashion in the supine position with a bump under the ipsilateral ischium.[1,7] A 5-cm anterior incision is used to expose the Smith-Peterson interval (tensor fascia lata [TFL] laterally and the sartorius medially). After retracting the exposed rectus femoris muscle medially and cauterizing the lateral femoral circumflex vessels, the anterior hip capsule is exposed (**Figure 1**). Hohmann retractors are placed around the femoral neck, and the hip capsule is incised along the length of the femoral neck from the acetabulum to the intertrochanteric line. The capsule is retracted superiorly and inferiorly. The level of the femoral osteotomy is confirmed under c-arm fluoroscopy and the cut is made under direct vision (**Figure 2**). The acetabulum is exposed with the use of three Hohmann retractors (**Figure 3**). After excising the labrum, the acetabulum is reamed to 45° of abduction and 20° of anteversion. An uncemented acetabular component is then impacted into place and its position confirmed under fluoroscopy (**Figure 4**). Because of a tendency to slightly over-antevert the acetabular component, some surgeons choose to place a 10° elevated polyethylene liner with the maximal buildup anteriorly.

Attention is then turned to the placement of the femoral component. A second 3.8- to 5-cm posterior incision is made in the buttock and the gluteus maximus fibers are split to locate the piriformis fossa (**Figure 5**). To facilitate the exposure, the operative extremity is adducted and placed in neutral rotation. An awl is placed into the femoral canal through this incision

FIGURE 1

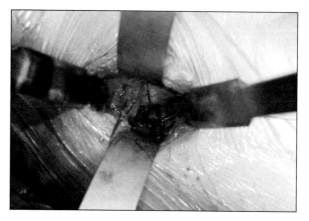

Smith-Peterson approach to the femoral neck. The rectus femoris is retracted medially, exposing the capsule and the fat pad overlying the femoral neck.

under fluoroscopic guidance. Sequential reamers and broaches are used under close fluoroscopic guidance to widen the canal to the appropriate size. A fully coated diaphyseal engaging femoral stem has been recommended with this two-incision technique. Developers of the two-incision LIS-THA found that preparation of the diaphyseal bone with sequentially larger straight reamers was more reliable and reproducible than was preparation of the metaphyseal bone for a proximally coated stem. Broaches are seated with a combination of fluoroscopic guidance and direct visualization through the anterior incision. A trial neck and head is placed on the appropriately sized broach and range of motion and stability are evaluated under direct and fluoroscopic visualization. The femoral component is placed through the posterior incision and impacted until it is within 1 cm of the calcar. Longitudinal traction is applied to the leg, and the neck of the implant is pulled through the posterior soft tissues and into the acetabulum. The femoral component is then observed through the anterior incision to confirm appropriate anteversion as final seating of the implant is done (**Figure 6**). Trial reduction is performed to choose the femoral head that best restores leg length and offset.

After placement of the real femoral head, the incisions are irrigated and the anterior capsule is closed with interrupted sutures. The fascia and the skin of both incisions are closed and a postoperative dressing is applied.

**FIGURE 2**

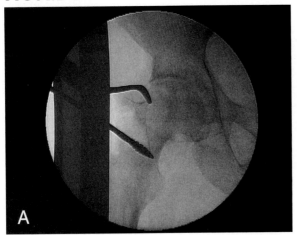
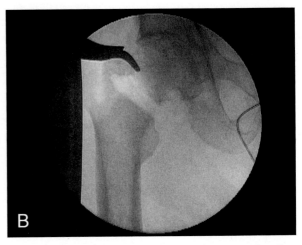

Femoral osteotomies. **A,** The first distal cut is made in the distal portion of the femoral neck under direct vision using fluoroscopy confirmation. A second proximal cut is made approximately 2 cm above the first cut and is aimed slightly distally and posteriorly to avoid the posterior acetabulum. This creates a 2-cm wedge that is slightly tapered from anterior to posterior and can be removed without difficulty. **B,** A fluoroscopic view of the proximal femur after both cuts have been made and the wedge is removed.

## SURGICAL PITFALLS AND COMMON ERRORS

### Initial Exposure of the Femoral Neck and Acetabulum

Finding and remaining in the proper interval with the Smith-Peterson approach is important. Flexing the hip better delineates this interval between the TFL and the sartorius. The underlying rectus femoris is exposed by making a small fascial incision over the TFL and digitally dissecting on the lateral side of the sartorius. This decreases the likelihood of injuring the lateral femoral cutaneous nerve.

A second pitfall occurs when surgeons inadvertently dissect down to the hip capsule medial to the rectus femoris. This mistake can be limited by preventing external rotation of the limb, which predisposes one to dissect on the medial side of the rectus.

### Femoral Neck Osteotomy and Acetabular Preparation

It is recommended that the femoral neck osteotomy be done with a series of cuts. The first cut should be in the proximal portion of the femoral neck aimed distally and posteriorly to avoid the posterior acetabulum. Then a more distal cut is made to create a 2-cm wedge that is slightly tapered from anterior to posterior to facilitate subsequent removal (**Figure 2**). After removing this wedge, the remaining femoral head is extracted as one piece. To prevent too low of a femoral cut, the second cut should be made under fluoroscopic guidance. The height of the femoral neck cut can be judged relative to the lesser trochanter in accordance with the preoperative plan. Any residual lateral bone spikes should be removed with a burr or a vertical cut using the saw with the hip held in abduction and mild traction.

When preparing the acetabulum, it is important to recognize the limitation of the anterior exposure. The posterior capsule tends to aggregate near the inferior aspect of the acetabulum where one might expect to find the transverse acetabular ligament; however, this portion of the posterior capsule should not be excised. Surgeons should be aware of the tendency to ream and place the acetabular component in an excessively anteverted and excessively vertical position. Intraoperative fluoroscopy can be used to evaluate acetabular component placement. Using as a reference an imaginary line connecting the radiographic teardrop of each acetabulum, the surgeon aims to place the acetabular component to

**FIGURE 3**

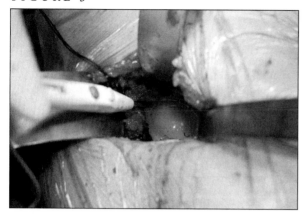

After removing the femoral neck following the osteotomy, the acetabulum is exposed with the use of three Hohmann retractors.

**FIGURE 4**

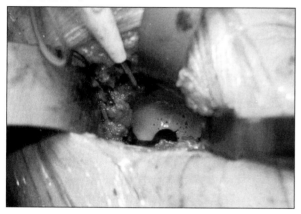

The acetabulum is prepared with reaming to 45° of abduction and 20° of anteversion until healthy bleeding is seen through the acetabulum. A cementless acetabular component is then impacted into place and its position confirmed under fluoroscopy.

achieve a lateral opening (vertical position) that does not exceed 45° relative to that line. Some surgeons choose to place two screws in the acetabulum because of the possibility of dislodgement of the acetabular component during placement of the real femoral component.

## Femoral Preparation and Implant Insertion

Preparation of the femoral canal and placement of the femoral component through the posterior incision is aided by the use of fluoroscopy. It is important to protect the posterior soft tissues when placing the awl, reamers, and broaches into this area. These sharp instruments cause measurable muscle damage. Insertion of the femoral component often is the most challenging part of the operation. Cautery or a knife should be used to incise the posterosuperior joint capsule to allow passage of the real implant. The collar and trunion on the real femoral component make it substantially more difficult to insert than the broaches. The trunion often has a tendency to catch on the posterosuperior part of the acetabulum and be pushed into excessive anteversion. The anteversion of the stem should be checked directly through the anterior incision prior to final seating.

## POSTOPERATIVE CARE

### Pain Management

**Inpatient**

At our institution, patients undergoing traditional or minimally invasive THA are placed on a multimodal total joint regional analgesia pathway.[8] This pathway uses multiple modalities to lessen a patient's need for intravenous narcotic pain medication. A major goal of this pathway is to facilitate rapid rehabilitation while avoiding the unwanted side effects of narcotics such as nausea, constipation, pruritis, and urinary retention.

Another aim of the total joint regional analgesia pathway is to provide preemptive analgesia. This is defined as the administration of pain medication prior to the surgical insult and prior to the development of marked postoperative pain. These principles have been derived from studies demonstrating that patients often require large doses and rapid administration of narcotic medication once the pain had become intolerable. Scheduled administration of oxycodone and acetaminophen at our institution has greatly decreased the need for both intravenous and oral narcotic medication postoperatively.[9]

Preoperatively, patients receive acetaminophen, a nonsteroidal anti-inflammatory drug, and a long-acting narcotic medication. The mainstay of the total joint regional analgesia pathway, however, is a peripheral nerve block. Total hip arthroplasty patients receive a psoas compartment block of the lumbar plexus using an indwelling catheter prior to entering the operating room. Alterna-

## FIGURE 5

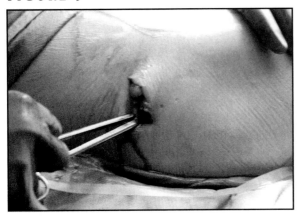

A second 3.8- to 5-cm posterior incision is made in the buttock to find the interval between the abductor and external rotator muscles. The piriformis tendon can be palpated and the interval identified just superior to the piriformis. The starting point for reaming is similar to that for a closed femoral nailing.

## FIGURE 6

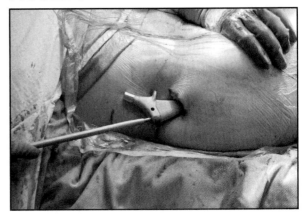

The femoral canal is reamed under fluoroscopic guidance and then broached. The femoral component is then placed through the posterior incision and impacted until it is within 1 cm of the calcar. Longitudinal traction is then applied to the leg and the neck of the implant is pulled through the posterior soft tissues and into the acetabulum. The femoral component is then observed through the anterior incision to confirm appropriate anteversion prior to final seating.

tively, a fascia iliaca block can be done, but the block does not reliably cover the lateral femoral cutaneous or obturator nerves.

A short-acting spinal anesthetic is given to provide complete pain relief during the surgery itself. Postoperatively, patients are given acetaminophen, ketorolac, and a long-acting narcotic medication on a schedule rather than on an "as needed" basis. The indwelling psoas catheter is left in place, and the infusion of the local anesthetic is slowly titrated over the first postoperative day and discontinued on the morning of the second postoperative day. This usually encompasses the postoperative period when the patient would otherwise require intravenous narcotics; by the time the indwelling catheter is discontinued, the patient is tolerating a regular diet and can take oral pain medications on a scheduled basis to maintain good pain control (preemptive analgesia).

### Outpatient

The study by Berger and associates[5] indicated that surgery can be performed using an epidural catheter and a short-acting sedative. If this is done as the first case of the operative day, the patient can be monitored on the orthopaedic floor after the removal of the epidural catheter approximately 4 hours after surgery. The patient

is given a long-acting oral narcotic (oxycodone 20 mg PO 2 hours after surgery) and can be given intravenous pain medication as needed. Patients are transitioned to oral analgesic medications alone by the evening of surgery. Discharge can be considered once the pain is controlled well with oral medication alone.

## Physical Therapy

### Outpatient

In addition to aggressive postoperative pain management to facilitate discharge of patients on the same day as surgery, patients must complete physical therapy. In the outpatient protocol,[5] occupational and physical therapy are initiated approximately 6 hours after surgery. Patients are weight bearing as tolerated on the operative extremity and therapy starts with the patient transferring from the bed to a chair. Once this is completed, the patient walks with crutches, first with the assistance of a physical therapist and then without. Patients are then taught how to ascend and descend stairs using crutches, first with the assistance of a physical therapist and then without. After meeting these criteria, patients are considered ready for discharge to their homes.

**Inpatient**

At our institution, all patients are moved from the bed to a chair on the evening of surgery. Ambulation with a walker or crutches (with weight bearing as tolerated) is initiated on the morning of the first postoperative day.[4] Patients undergo two sessions of physical therapy daily during inpatient hospitalization. Patients are discharged from the hospital when they can get in and out of bed with minimal assistance, walk more than 50 feet with a walker or two crutches, walk up and down three steps, and require only oral medications for pain control. The walker or crutches are discontinued in favor of a cane when the patient feels comfortable. The patient is then slowly weaned from the cane at his or her discretion over the next few weeks.

# RESULTS

Interpretation of the clinical results of two-incision LIS-THA is best done by systematically reviewing: (1) the initial reports from surgeon-developers, (2) subsequent reports from non-developers, and (3) emerging data from direct comparison studies and randomized controlled trials. These findings are summarized in **Table 2**.

The first series of patients reported by Berger[1] in 2003 had excellent clinical results at short-term follow-up. The patients had no complications (with the exception of one intraoperative proximal femoral fracture), no dislocations, no reoperations, and no infections. Radiographic follow-up of 30 patients at 1 year showed bone ingrowth in all patients, with 91% of femoral stems placed between neutral and 3° of valgus.

Patients undergoing this procedure also rehabilitated very quickly and successfully.[5] All of the patients met hospital discharge criteria at 23 hours; and the last 88 patients in the study were offered the surgery on an outpatient basis, with 75% of these patients successfully discharged from the hospital on the evening of surgery. No patients were readmitted to the hospital and none had any complications at home. The functional outcome measures in these patients are shown in **Table 3**.

The combined results of a multicenter study involving 275 patients from Berry and associates[2] showed a slight increase in the prevalence of complications. The prevalence of major complications was determined to be 3.2%, with a minor complication rate of 8%. This consisted of two dislocations, three femoral fractures,

one femoral subsidence, three calcar fractures, two partial femoral nerve palsies, and sixteen lateral femoral cutaneous nerve palsies. However, 82% of these patients were discharged from the hospital within 24 hours.

These initial series from the surgeon-developers of the two-incision technique were certainly favorable in a selected group of patients.[1,2,5,6] However, the advancements used to optimize these patient outcomes extend well beyond minimally invasive two-incision surgical techniques alone. In those studies, the surgeons also used preoperative patient education, comprehensive postoperative pain management techniques, and advanced physical therapy/rehabilitation protocols. Each of those measures can be important in improving patient outcomes and facilitating recovery. Thus, these initial developer reports do not provide sufficient evidence to prove that the observed benefits are attributable to the two-incision surgical technique itself.

When the two-incision technique was released to a wide range of surgeons, the prevalence of complications rose and a substantial learning curve was identified. The largest study assessing the effect of surgeon experience on the prevalence of complications in two-incision LIS-THA was performed by Archibeck and White.[10] This study assessed the experience of 159 surgeons with 851 total cases and noted that increased surgeon experience led to decreased blood loss, shorter surgical times, and a lower prevalence of femoral fracture. Lateral femoral cutaneous nerve palsies were present in only 3.2% of patients. The study concluded that complications are most likely to be associated with surgeons who have performed less than 10 two-incision LIS-THAs, with surgeons who perform less than 50 total hip arthroplasties per year, and when the surgery is performed on obese patients (BMI > 30 kg/m$^2$).

Mardones and associates[3] conducted a cadaver study to assess the contention that the two-incision LIS-THA could be done without damage to any muscle or tendon around the hip. Ten cadavers were obtained and a two-incision LIS-THA was performed on one hip by an experienced surgeon. On the contralateral hip, a mini-posterior THA was performed. The amount of muscle damage to the gluteus medius and minimus was determined by gross examination by an independent observer. Every two-incision THA had measurable damage to the abductors, the external rotators, or both. Furthermore, the two-incision technique resulted in greater

TABLE 2

## Surgical Data and Rate of Complications in the Large Series of Two-incision Less Invasive Total Hip Arthroplasties

| Study | Overall Rate of Complications | Major Complication Rate | Minor Complication Rate | Reoperation Rate | Average Estimated Blood Loss (mL) | Average Surgical Time (min) | Pertinent Findings |
|---|---|---|---|---|---|---|---|
| Berger (2003) | 1% | 1% | 0% | 0% | Not Reported | 106 | 100% of patients discharged within 3 days. Of the last 88 patients, 85% went home the same day, 15% home postoperative day 1. |
| Mears, et al (2003) | 11.2% | 3.2% | 8% | 0.4% | Not Reported | 78.5 | 82% discharged with-in 24 hours. |
| Archibeck & White (2004) | 12.5% | 10% | 2% | 1% | 496 | 148 | Decreased rate of complications with surgeons who perform 450 THAs per year. |
| Pagnano, et al (2005) | 39% | 14% | 25% | 5% | Not Reported | 68 | Mean hospitalization= 2.8 days. 90% of patients discharged home. |
| Bal, et al (2005) | 42% | 13% | 29% | 10% | 545 | 127 | Decreased rate of major complications with surgeon experience. No change in rate of minor complications. |

damage to the gluteus medius muscle and the gluteus minimus muscle when compared to the mini-posterior approach (**Figure 7**).

Our group retrospectively reviewed 80 consecutive patients at the Mayo Clinic who underwent two-incision LIS-THA.[4] These patients had longer average surgical times when compared to patients undergoing THA via the standard posterior approach. This longer surgical time was not reduced with surgeon experience; patients late in the series had similar surgical times to patients early in the series. The prevalence of complications was also greater in the two-incision group, with a major complication rate of 14% (compared to 5% in the standard posterior approach group). These complications included four intraoperative calcar fractures, three postoperative femoral fractures, two femoral nerve palsies,

FIGURE 7

A) Gluteus Medius Muscle

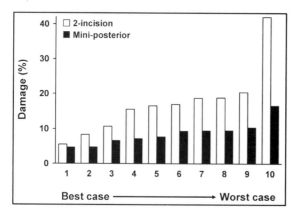

B) Gluteus Medius Tendon

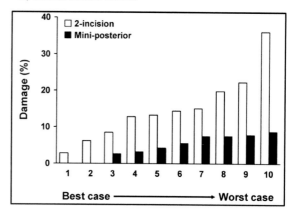

C) Gluteus Minimus Muscle

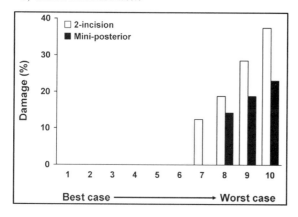

D) Gluteus Minimus Tendon

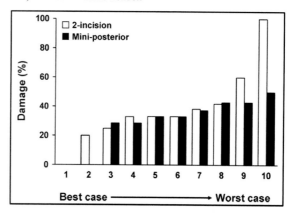

Diagrams showing the level of muscle/tendon injury in cadavers when comparing two-incision less invasive total hip arthroplasty with the minimally invasive posterior approach. Cases are listed from 1 (best case) through 10 (worst case): (A) Gluteus medius muscle, (B) Gluteus medius tendon, (C) Gluteus minimus muscle, and (D) Gluteus minimus tendon. *(Printed with permission from Mardones R, Pagnano MW, Nemanich JP, Trousdale RT: The Frank Stinchfield Award: Muscle damage after total hip arthroplasty done with the two-incision and mini-posterior techniques. Clin Orthop Relat Res 2005;441:63-67).*

one femoral subsidence, and one recurrent dislocation. Interestingly, these complications were not limited to patients treated early in the series; complications were seen throughout the series of 80 patients. Older, obese women (BMI > 30 kg/m$^2$) were identified as having a higher risk of major complications than the average patient and the same patient treated with a standard posterior approach. The prevalence of reoperation was also higher in the two-incision group (5% compared to 1% in the standard posterior approach group). The

functional outcome measures for these patients are shown in **Table 3**.

The study of Bal and associates[11] on 89 hips with two-incision LIS-THA indicated a 42% prevalence of complications in the two-incision group (compared to 6% in the single-incision group). The major complications were largely responsible for the 10% reoperation rate; two patients had postoperative femoral fractures, five had intraoperative femoral fractures, four had femoral subsidence/loosening, and one had recurrent disloca-

**TABLE 3**

**Comparison of Functional Outcome Measures in Two Series of Patients**

|  | Mayo | Berger |
|---|---|---|
| Average time to discharge | 2.8 days | 20 hours |
| Percent discharged home | 90% | 100% |
| Time to discontinuation of narcotics | 9 days | 6 days |
| Time to discontinuation of crutches | 14 days | 6 days |
| Time to resuming driving | 6 weeks | 6 days |
| Return to work | 8 weeks | 8 days |
| Resume daily activities | 14 days | 10 days |
| Discontinued use of cane | 28 days | 14 days |

tions. Most of the other complications were minor, with thigh numbness the most common problem (25% of patients). The authors concluded that the strikingly high rate of complications did not justify the two-incision procedure (**Table 2**).

Interestingly, this study also assessed the surgeons' ability to decrease the rate of complications with experience. The first 40 patients were compared to the last 49 patients. The number of overall complications decreased from 55% to 31%, whereas major complications reduced from 33% to 4%. However, the proportion of patients with thigh numbness remained stable, from 23% in the first group to 27% in the second group.

Pagnano and associates[12] studied a series of 26 patients who had staged bilateral total hip arthroplasties with a less invasive two-incision technique performed on one side and a mini-posterior technique on the other side. The same comprehensive anesthesia and rapid rehabilitation protocols were used after each THA. All patients had a successful outcome with no complications after either hip. At 6 months after the second THA, patients were reviewed. There were no differences in time to discontinuation of ambulatory aids, return to driving, climbing stairs, return to work, or walking ½ mile. Sixteen of 26 patients preferred the mini-posterior hip based on a perceived quicker or easier recovery compared to the two-incision hip.

The most comprehensive analysis of the two-incision technique was recently reported. Pagnano and associates[13] performed a prospective randomized trial of two-incision LIS-THA versus mini-posterior THA and sought to: (1) determine if patients recovered faster after two-incision THA than after mini-posterior THA as determined by functional milestones that reflect activities of daily living; (2) determine if the clinical outcome after two-incision THA was better than that after mini-posterior THA as measured by SF-12 scores; and (3) evaluate the technical difficulties of the two-incision THA compared to mini-posterior THA as judged by the surgical time and the prevalence of complications.

A computerized randomization process dynamically balanced the groups based on age, gender, race, and BMI. Seventy-two patients with a mean age of 66 years and a mean BMI of 30 were enrolled and this included 20 men and 16 women in each group. The two-incision patients recovered more slowly than the mini-posterior patients as measured by the mean time to discontinue crutches, to discontinue all ambulatory aids, and to return to normal daily activities. The clinical outcome as measured by SF-12 scores was similar in both groups at both 2 months and 1 year postoperatively. The two-incision THA was technically more difficult with a mean surgical time that was 24 minutes longer than the mini-posterior THA. The prevalence of complications was the same between the groups (2.4%). This prospective, randomized trial dispels the notion that the two-incision THA technique improves short-term recovery after THA. Instead, it was the mini-posterior patients who had the quicker recovery.

## CONCLUSION

Since 2002, the introduction of two-incision LIS-THA has changed the field of hip arthroplasty. It has done so by bringing to surgeons' attention the importance of patient education, improved pain control, and the benefits of well-organized early physical therapy protocols. However, there is no scientific evidence to date that the two-incision LIS-THA technique itself is safer, more efficient, or improves patient outcomes more effectively than other minimally invasive or conventional methods.

The claim that two-incision LIS-THA causes less damage to muscles and tendons has been studied in cadaveric hips.[3] Evaluation of the gluteus medius and minimus muscles demonstrated increased damage via the two-incision approach compared to the mini-posterior approach. The demonstrated damage to the external rotators (piriformis and conjoined tendon) in the two-incision technique was surprising as well. Functional tests and gait analysis tests of patients who have undergone two-incision LIS-THA are necessary to determine the clinical importance of this muscle damage. Regardless, it is apparent that the two-incision technique does not lead to decreased damage to the hip musculature.

Multiple studies performed since 2002 have demonstrated a high number of complications when compared with conventional total hip arthroplasty. The most common major complications are intraoperative calcar fractures, femoral neck fractures, femoral subsidence, and recurrent dislocation. These were largely responsible for the increased reoperation rate in patients undergoing two-incision LIS-THA. Whereas most of the complications are minor (such as lateral femoral cutaneous injury), the frequency of these is alarming and the rate does not appear to diminish with increased surgeon expertise. Moreover, these complications (both major and minor) are observed much less often in patients treated via a standard posterior approach.

The discrepancy in the data among the various studies may be attributed not only to surgeon experience, but also to differences in patient populations. For example, the average age of the patients in Berger's[1] series of 100 patients was 55 years, 75% of the subjects were men, and the average patient weight was 80 kg. In contrast, the Mayo Clinic experience consisted of patients with an average age of 70.5 years, 56% of the subjects were women, and the average patient weight was 93 kg. Thus, it is apparent that patient differences may play a role in the wide differences in the rate of complications and the rate of recovery. Some clear trends noted in multiple studies proved to be predictors of poor outcomes in patients undergoing two-incision LIS-THA. The three most clearly identified predictors of poor outcomes are female gender, older age, and obesity (BMI > 30 kg/m$^2$).

Attempting to correct for patient differences and provide a fair comparison of two-incision LIS-THA to a standard approach to THA can be difficult. One recent study looked at patients who had one hip replaced with the two-incision technique and the other replaced via a mini-posterior approach. In that study, most patients preferred the mini-posterior approach and the most common reason was that the mini-posterior approach allowed an easier recovery. Cosmesis was not improved with the two-incision technique.

Minimally invasive techniques furthered by advances in technology will play a role in the future of total joint reconstructive surgery. However, these techniques need to be subjected to rigorous laboratory, clinical, and functional testing in the short- and mid-term prior to advocating them to patients with confidence. At this point, we can state with clarity that: (1) there is no scientific evidence that the two-incision technique is better than other approaches to THA in comparable groups of patients; (2) for many surgeons the prevalence of complications with the two-incision technique is high; and (3) the procedure cannot be done routinely without measurable muscle damage. At our institution we have been disappointed with the two-incision technique for the typical THA patient; the added difficulty has not been rewarded with better functional results or better cosmetic results.

## REFERENCES

1. Berger RA: Total hip arthroplasty using the minimally invasive two-incision approach. *Clin Orthop Relat Res* 2003;417:232-241.

2. Berry DJ, Berger RA, Callaghan JJ, et al: Minimally invasive total hip arthroplasty: Development, early results, and a critical analysis. Presented at the Annual Meeting of the American Orthopaedic Association, Charleston, South Carolina, USA, June 14, 2003. *J Bone Joint Surg Am* 2003;85:2235-2246.

3. Mardones R, Pagnano MW, Nemanich JP, Trousdale RT: The Frank Stinchfield Award: Muscle damage after total hip arthroplasty done with the two-incision and mini-posterior techniques. *Clin Orthop Relat Res* 2005;441:63-67.

4. Pagnano MW, Leone J, Lewallen DG, Hanssen AD: Two-incision THA had modest outcomes and some substantial complications. *Clin Orthop Relat Res* 2005;441:86-90.

5. Berger RA, Jacobs JJ, Meneghini RM, Della Valle C, Paprosky W, Rosenberg AG: Rapid rehabilitation and recovery with minimally invasive total hip arthroplasty. *Clin Orthop Relat Res* 2004;429:239-247.

6. Berger RA: Mini-incisions: Two for the price of one! *Orthopedics* 2002;25:472-498.

7. Berger RA, Duwelius PJ: The two-incision minimally invasive total hip arthroplasty: Technique and results. *Orthop Clin North Am* 2004;35:163-172.

8. Hebl JR, Kopp SL, Ali MH, et al: A comprehensive anesthesia protocol that emphasizes peripheral nerve blockade for total knee and total hip arthroplasty. *J Bone Joint Surg Am* 2005;87:63-70.

9. Horlocker TT, Kopp SL, Pagnano MW, Hebl JR: Analgesia for total hip and knee arthroplasty: A multimodal pathway featuring peripheral nerve block. *J Am Acad Orthop Surg* 2006;14:126-135.

10. Archibeck MJ, White RE Jr: Learning curve for the two-incision total hip replacement. *Clin Orthop Relat Res* 2004;429:232-238.

11. Bal BS, Haltom D, Aleto T, Barrett M: Early complications of primary total hip replacement performed with a two-incision minimally invasive technique. *J Bone Joint Surg Am* 2005;87:2432-2438.

12. Pagnano MW, Trousdale RT, Meneghini RM, Hanssen AD: Patients preferred a mini-posterior THA to a contralateral two-incision THA. *Clin Orthop Relat Res* 2006, Sept 21 (Epub ahead of print.)

13. Pagnano MW, Trousdale RT, Leone J, Meneghini RM, Hanssen AD: A prospective randomized trial shows that two-incision total hips do not recover quicker than mini-posterior total hips. Presented at 16th Annual Meeting American Association of Hip and Knee Surgeons, Dallas, Texas, November 2006.

# CHAPTER 3

# LIMITED INCISION MUSCLE-SPARING ANTEROLATERAL WATSON-JONES APPROACH FOR TOTAL HIP ARTHROPLASTY

KENNETH GUSTKE, MD

Total hip arthroplasty (THA) without the need for postoperative restrictions is one of the most desirable situations for both the patient and the surgeon. Having no restrictions and adequate postoperative pain control provide the best potential for faster rehabilitation. With mini- and standard incision THA techniques, some muscle is detached for exposure and needs time to heal. Therefore, most surgeons restrict postoperative weight bearing, range of motion, and delay the onset of resistive exercises.[1-3] The ideal limited incision approach would be when no muscle is detached, therefore resulting in no postoperative restrictions.

A minimally invasive modification of the Watson-Jones approach was conceived by Heinz Roettinger, MD from Munich, Germany in 2003.[4] In this muscle-sparing approach, a single 8- to 12-cm incision is used anterior and proximal to the greater trochanter. The acetabulum and proximal femur are exposed through a single window in the intermuscular interval between the gluteus medius and tensor fascia lata. No fluoroscopy is needed. The abductors and posterior capsule are not detached, eliminating violation of the structures that

may lead to weakness with standard and smaller incision Hardinge direct lateral with detachment and subsequent repair of a portion of the abductor muscles and dislocations with the posterior approach with detachment and subsequent repair of the external rotators. Using this modification, there is no need to restrict postoperative range of motion or weight bearing, and resistive exercises can be started earlier. Total time for recovery is influenced mainly by the time needed to strengthen atrophied muscles.

All patients are potential candidates for this modified Watson-Jones approach, although patients with coxa vara deformities and very muscular men are more difficult to treat. Obese patients are difficult to treat no matter what surgical approach is used. However, since there is usually less underlying adipose tissue anterior than directly lateral or posterior, the limited incision anterolateral approach appears to be less difficult than others.

## PREOPERATIVE PATIENT EDUCATION

All preoperative patients are provided a monograph on the surgical procedure, which includes a description of the surgical procedure, expected benefits, risks, and possible complications. Also included is a list of gentle nonresistive range-of-motion exercises that the patient is requested to try to perform. A preoperative home visit from a physical therapist includes a review of the use of a walker and cane, and assessment for adverse home situations.

## SURGICAL TECHNIQUE

The patient is placed on the operating table in the lateral decubitus position using a rigid pelvic positioner. The table is modified either with an L-shaped wooden or plastic extension or special table extension such that the posterior half of the table beyond the pelvis is absent. This modification is required to place the leg in an extended, adducted, and externally rotated position for the femoral preparation (**Figure 1**). Placing the patient obliquely on a standard operating table does not allow adequate hip adduction during femoral preparation.

An 8- to 12-cm incision is made along the anterior greater trochanter, extending anteriorly and proximally over the underlying palpable anterior border of the gluteus medius (**Figure 2**). The proximal limb of the incision should aim between the anterior superior iliac spine and the gluteal tubercle. Too anterior placement of the incision should be avoided so as not to damage the anterior femoral cutaneous nerve. The fascia is incised in the line of the incision. The gluteus medius is immediately visible under the proximal half of the fascial incision. Distally, the interval between the gluteus medius and tensor fascia lata is more apparent because they begin to diverge in direction. The interval is opened 2 to 3 cm in a proximal direction to avoid injury to the superior gluteal nerve branch to the tensor fascia lata (**Figure 3**). With the femur slightly abducted, finger dissection proximally along the anterior trochanter will take one down to the femoral neck and anterolaterally under the gluteus medius and minimus. A retractor is inserted between the gluteus minimus and the capsule. Another retractor is placed anteriorly between the rectus femoris and the capsule (**Figure 4**). These retractors are specially designed with broad curved surfaces to lessen point pressure on the muscles, and they are also lit to add visualization. The anterior capsule is incised with either a T- or Z-shaped incision (**Figure 5**). The retractors are reinserted inside the capsule, exposing the femoral neck and base of the head (**Figure 6**). With the femur maximally

externally rotated, the femoral neck is osteotomized at the subcapital level (**Figure 7**). The neck is then levered up (**Figure 8**), the femur is fully externally rotated, and the leg is placed perpendicular to the floor in a sterile drape bag off the posterior side of the table. The junction of the lateral femoral neck and medial greater trochanter is identified. This area is referred to as the "saddle" (**Figure 8**). Because the lesser trochanter is not visible or palpable at this point, the saddle becomes the landmark for the distal femoral neck osteotomy based on preoperative templating (**Figure 9**). The osteotomized neck fragment is removed. The femur can now be flexed, abducted, and externally rotated for visualization of the lesser trochanter. The neck length for the cut can be confirmed or adjusted if the lesser trochanter is used for preoperative planning.

The thigh and leg are slightly abducted and externally rotated on top of the contralateral leg. The proximal femur is retracted posterior and inferior to the acetabulum. Another retractor is placed along the anteroinferior acetabulum, retracting the anteromedial capsule (**Figure 10**). An additional retractor may be placed superiorly to retract the anterolateral capsule. The femoral head fragment is removed from the acetabulum (**Figure 11**). An excellent straight-on view of the entire acetabulum should be present (**Figure 12**). The acetabulum is prepared in a customary fashion. Using side cut-out reamer heads and a curved reamer handle lessens soft-tissue irritation on insertion and allows reaming at a normal abduction and anteversion angle (**Figure 13**). Use of a curved shell impactor facilitates acetabular component positioning through a shorter skin incision distally. The acetabular shell is inserted using an alignment rod pointing to the center of the shoulder (**Figure 14**). Screws may be used if necessary. A standard non-lipped acetabular liner is now inserted. Any remaining acetabular osteophytes are removed.

For femoral preparation, the leg is externally rotated, adducted, and extended into a drape pocket in the space where the posterior half of the distal part of the table was removed. One retractor is placed over the tip of the greater trochanter to retract the anterior gluteus medius. Another retractor is placed under the posterior medial neck to elevate the neck (**Figure 15**). Any remaining capsule attached to the lateral neck is released back to the piriformis fossa. This capsular release facilitates better neck elevation into the surgical field (**Figure 16**). If the

**FIGURE 1**

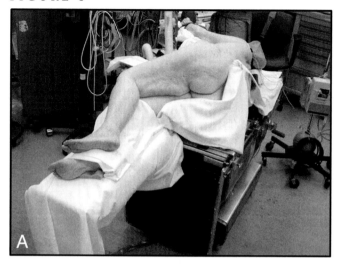
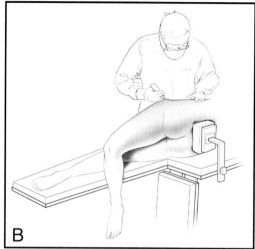

**A,** Laminated wood table extension. **B,** During femoral preparation, the leg is extended, adducted, and externally rotated into the removed area posterior. (Obtained with permission: Zimmer Orthopedics)

**FIGURE 2**

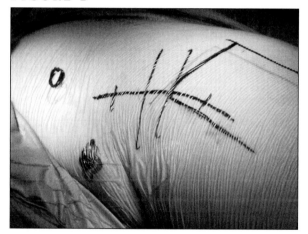

An 8- to 12-cm incision is made along the anterior greater trochanter and over the underlying anterior border of the gluteus medius. The superior limb aims between the anterior superior iliac spine and the gluteal tubercle.

femoral component preparation requires femoral canal sizing or reaming, a sleeve is used around the reamer shaft to protect the proximal soft tissue (**Figure 17**). An anatomic shaped femoral component broach does not require a special broach or implant handle modification because its curve eases insertion without proximal soft-tissue impingement (**Figure 18**). Straight stems can be

**FIGURE 3**

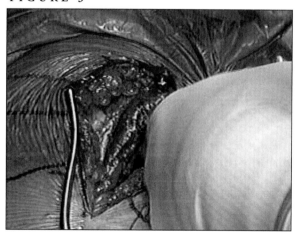

The interval between the gluteus medius and tensor fascia is opened.

used with special offset broach and implant handles. Broaching is performed until stability is achieved. Calcar planing is performed for collared implants. A trial reduction is performed (the hip is placed into positions of hyperextension/adduction/external rotation, flexion/adduction/internal rotation, and abduction/flexion/external rotation to check for instability or impingement). Correct leg lengths are confirmed with the overlay leg method or with computer navigation. The

FIGURE 4

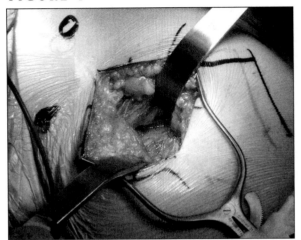

The joint capsule is exposed with retraction of the gluteus medius and minimus laterally and the tensor fascia lata and rectus femoris medially.

FIGURE 5

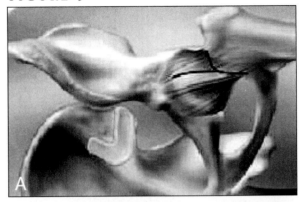

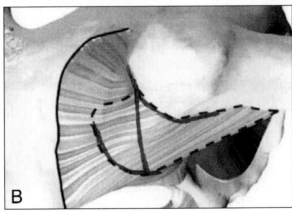

**A,** Use of a T-shaped capsulotomy. **B,** A Z-shaped capsulotomy provides a wider exposure but it is more difficult to repair the superior limb later.

definitive femoral component and head are then inserted and the hip is reduced (**Figure 19**).

Closure is simple because no detached muscle needs to be repaired. The vertical part of the T- or Z-capsulotomy incision is closed, followed by the fascia, subcutaneous tissue, and skin.

## PITFALLS

There are several pitfalls to avoid. The lesser trochanter cannot be palpated until the femoral neck osteotomy fragment is removed. The best initial anatomic landmark for the more distal neck osteotomy is the "saddle," which is at the junction of the lateral femoral neck and the medial greater trochanter. Preoperative radiographic templating should reference the level of the distal femoral osteotomy to this anatomic point. After the neck fragment is removed, confirmation of the appropriate level cut level can then be determined relative to the lesser trochanter with abduction, external rotation, and flexion of the limb.

Inadequate acetabular exposure may occur if insufficient femoral neck is not initially removed. As much femoral neck as appropriate should be removed initially. It is important to relax tension on the anterior and posterior acetabular retractors after placing the acetabular component into position and before impaction. The tendency is for the assistant to place excessive force on the

posterior acetabular retractor which results in movement of the acetabulum into a more retroverted position. If the acetabular shell is now inserted, an unexpected increased anteverted position of the acetabular component can occur.

In very muscular patients, it may be difficult to displace the proximal femur up away from the acetabulum. It is important to make sure the lateral capsule is incised from the lateral neck to the piriformis fossa. If the capsule is still attached in this area, it can be palpated while the proximal femur is elevated with a bone hook. Occasionally, a tight piriformis may also require release. This is usually seen in patients with acetabular protrusio or with a severe external rotation contracture.

Since the tip of the greater trochanter is not visible, there is a tendency to insert the femoral component in varus. It is important to remove any remaining lateral

FIGURE 6

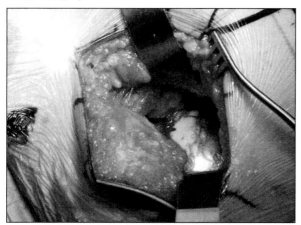

Exposed femoral neck.

FIGURE 7

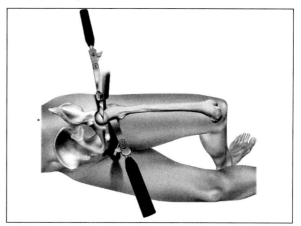

Proximal femoral neck osteotomy. (Obtained with permission: Zimmer Orthopedics)

FIGURE 8

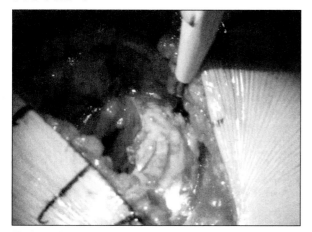

The femoral neck is dislocated from the head. The cautery tip is at the saddle.

FIGURE 9

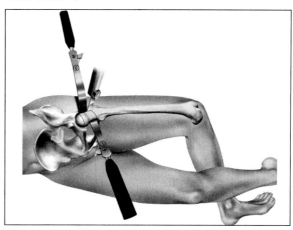

Osteotomy of the distal femoral neck. (Obtained with permission: Zimmer Orthopedics)

neck that would force the broach into varus. Also, if a broach much smaller than what had been preoperatively templated for appears stable, make sure it is not varus positioned. Rarely intraoperative radiographs may be needed to confirm appropriate broach positioning if in doubt.

The proper position of the ipsilateral leg dramatically improves visualization at each step. Therefore, it is important that the assistant is knowledgeable in leg positioning or that the surgeon continuously confirms the proper leg position (**Figure 20**). The surgery is more easily performed with two assistants; however, it can be per-formed with one assistant if the surgical scrub technician can assist periodically.

## CURRENT ANESTHESIA TECHNIQUE

Following completion of the study group surgeries, modifications in anesthesia have been instituted. Based on patient preference, the limited incision anterolateral patients receive either a spinal alone, a combination spinal and general anesthetic, or a general with a high femoral nerve catheter block. The spinal anesthetic provides better muscle relaxation than an epidural. Based on the patient's

## FIGURE 10

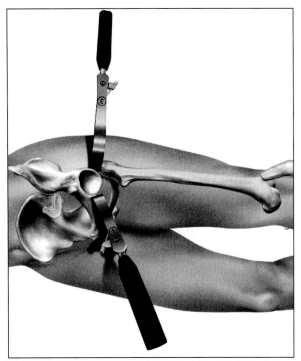

Exposure of the acetabulum. (Obtained with permission: Zimmer Orthopedics)

## FIGURE 11

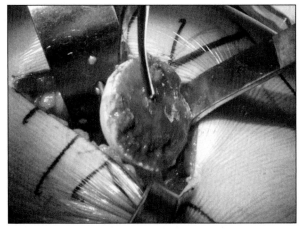

Removal of the femoral head.

size, 0.125 to 0.25 mg of morphine sulfate is inserted with the spinal anesthetic for postoperative pain relief. For the femoral block, a catheter is inserted as far proximally into the femoral nerve sheath to obtain a high lumbar block. For 36 hours, the patient controls the infusion of fentanyl citrate through this catheter via an infusion pump. A 4-mg dose of ondansetron is given intravenously 30 minutes before the end of the procedure to lessen postoperative nausea. Nonsteroidal analgesics and low-dose controlled release oxycodone are used for 36 to 48 hours.

## POSTOPERATIVE CARE

Physical therapy is started by at least the next morning. Some patients who underwent surgery in the morning may have physical therapy that same afternoon. Patients initially are placed on a walker and allowed weight bearing as tolerated. They begin range-of-motion exercises with no restrictions. Most patients are discharged to home on the second postoperative day. They are seen the following day, and three times weekly by a physical therapist in the home. When good balance is achieved, they are placed on a cane. This is usually within the first week postoperatively. As soon as their pain allows, they are started on resistive exercises. Patients desiring rapid muscle rehabilitation are referred to outpatient physical therapy between 2 and 3 weeks for more resistive exercises. The cane is discontinued when the patient can ambulate without a limp.

## RESULTS

The first 57 patients on which I performed this limited incision muscle-sparing anterolateral approach were compared to matched sets of total hips performed in 57 patients via a mini-incision direct lateral approach and in 57 patients via a standard incision direct lateral approach. The cases were matched by age, gender, diagnosis, body mass index, Charnley class, and bone type. Newer anesthesia techniques have been shown to improve recovery times. Purposely, no changes in anesthesia techniques were made on these groups of patients to bias the results and to determine the direct effect of the changes in surgical technique. Most patients received a combination general and spinal anesthetic. The limited incision anterolateral patients had no restrictions on weight bearing, range of motion, or the onset of resistive exercises. The mini- and standard direct lateral patients were requested to use partial weight bearing, and were allowed no hip flexion greater than 90° and no active hip abduction for 6 weeks. This was done in the later groups because of concerns about detachment of

**FIGURE 12**

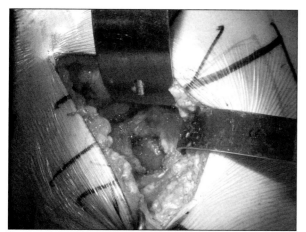

View of the acetabulum.

**FIGURE 13**

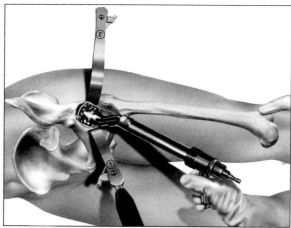

Use of a side cut-out reamer head and offset reamer handle facilitates insertion. (Obtained with permission: Zimmer Orthopedics)

**FIGURE 14**

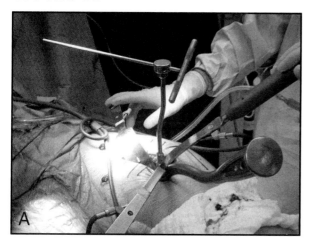

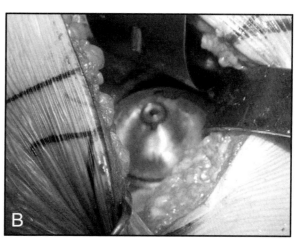

**A,** An offset shell inserter facilitates insertion and proper component positioning. **B,** The acetabular shell is in place. Screws can be inserted if necessary and any modular acetabular liner can be inserted.

the abductor muscle repair. The average incision length was 12.0 cm for the limited incision anterolateral patients, 11.0 for the mini-direct lateral patients, and 19.0 for the standard incision patients. The average surgical time was 116 minutes for the limited incision anterolateral patients, 113 minutes for the mini-direct lateral patients, and 127 minutes for the standard incision patients. The average hospital stay was 2.86 days for the limited incision anterolateral patients, 3.27 days for the mini-direct lateral patients, and 3.26 days for the standard incision patients. Patient-reported pain levels on a 0 to 10 scale were 37% less for the limited incision anterolateral group and 12% less for the mini-direct lateral group compared to the standard incision group for the first 3 days postoperatively. The mini-direct lateral and standard incision groups had essentially the same patient-reported pain levels at 2 and 6 weeks, whereas the limited incision anterolateral group had about 50%

FIGURE 15

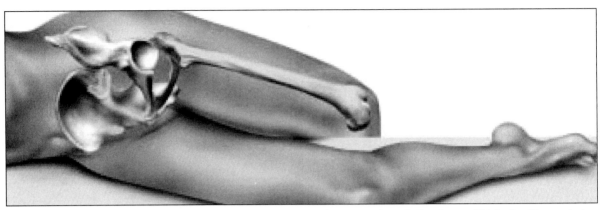

The ipsilateral leg is adducted, extended, and externally rotated for preparation of the femur. (Obtained with permission: Zimmer Orthopedics)

FIGURE 16

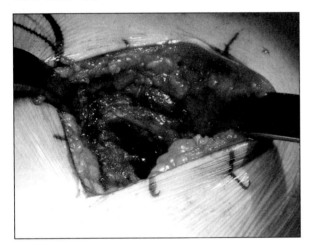

Proper visualization of the proximal femur.

FIGURE 17

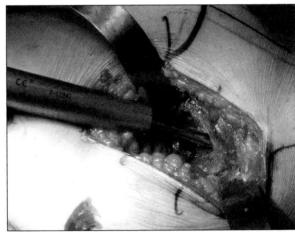

Soft-tissue protectors are used during femoral reaming.

less pain. The mini-direct lateral and standard incision patients could ambulate about the same distances during the first 3 days postoperatively, whereas the limited incision anterolateral patients could ambulate about two to five times further. The limited incision anterolateral patients began using a cane at an average of 12 days and discontinued use of the cane at an average of 25 days. Per our protocol, the mini-direct lateral and standard incision patients were recommended to continue use of a cane until a minimum of 90 days after surgery. No patients had lateral femoral cutaneous nerve injury-induced thigh numbness. There were no component malalignments, wound complications or infections, or dislocations in all groups. One of the limited incision anterolateral patients sustained a laceration of the profunda femoris artery, presumably from too inferior and medial placement of the inferior capsular retractor with a sharp tip. The hip arthroplasty was aborted and primary arterial repair was performed. Total hip arthroplasty was subsequently successfully performed about a month later via the limited incision anterolateral approach.

**FIGURE 18**

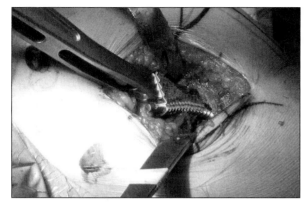

The handle on an anatomic stem broach does not impinge on soft tissue because of the curve on the proximal broach.

**FIGURE 19**

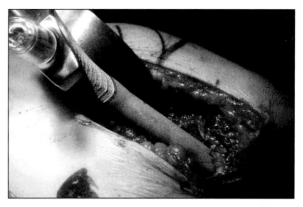

Insertion of an anatomic shaped femoral component. The hip is reduced.

**FIGURE 20**

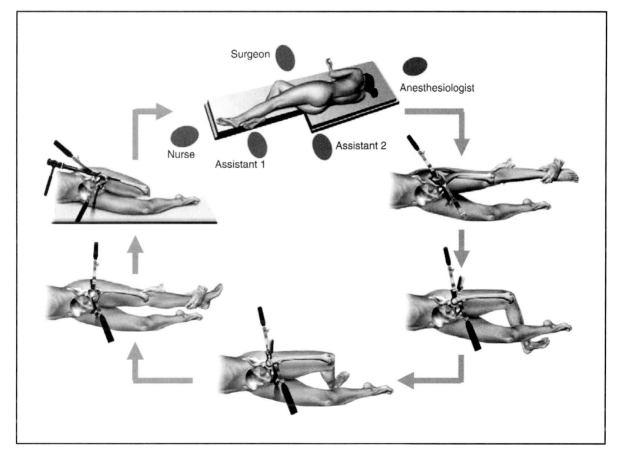

The assistant plays a very important role in manipulating the ipsilateral leg to optimize exposure. (Obtained with permission: Zimmer Orthopedics)

## Discussion and Conclusion

As my data shows, total hip arthroplasty performed via a limited incision muscle-sparing anterolateral Watson-Jones approach provides the potential short-term advantage of less initial pain than with a direct lateral approach via either a standard or mini-incision. The recovery curve is shifted toward more patients achieving faster recovery. The technique was safe and better, even in our early experience.

A frequent question about this intermuscular, but not internervous, approach is whether any patients sustain temporary or permanent denervation of the tensor fascia lata because of damage to the superior gluteal nerve branch that crosses the proximal side of the exposure interval. Electromyographic studies are now underway in several centers to answer this question. The tensor fascia lata is a hip abductor and pelvic stabilizer.[5] Clinically, these patients have demonstrated a return to excellent gait patterns and abductor muscle strength; if damage to the tensor fascia lata has occurred, it seems clinically insignificant.

Another unanswered question is whether the same results could be achieved with the mini-incision direct lateral and standard direct lateral approaches if no restrictions are placed on these patients. The literature and our personal experience leads us to believe that there may be a higher risk for dislocation and permanent abductor weakness if the standard direct lateral and mini-direct lateral patients are allowed no restrictions initially. This new technique will be an attractive alternative to other hip approaches, especially since most patients are candidates for this technique.

I have now performed this approach in over 250 patients. The incision length varies from 7 to 12 cm, depending on patient size. I use this approach for all primary total hip patients other than those with severe dysplasia or those requiring hardware removal from the femoral shaft.

## References

1. Kao JT, Woolson ST: Piriformis tendon repair failure after total hip replacement. *Orthop Rev* 1992;21:171-175.

2. Stahelin T, Vienne P, Hersche O: Failure of reinserted short external rotator muscles after total hip arthroplasty. *J Arthroplasty* 2002;17:604-607.

3. Svensson O, Skold S, Blomgren G: Integrity of the gluteus medius after the transgluteal approach in total hip arthroplasty. *J Arthroplasty* 1990;5:57-60.

4. Bertin KC, Rottinger H: Anterolateral mini-incision hip replacement surgery. *Clin Orthop Relat Res* 2004;429:248-255.

5. Gottschalk F, Kourosh S, Leveau B: The functional anatomy of tensor fasciae latae and gluteus medius and minimus. *J Anat* 1989;166:179-189.

# LIMITED INCISION DIRECT LATERAL TRANSMUSCULAR APPROACH FOR TOTAL HIP ARTHROPLASTY

GURDEEP S. BIRING, MSc, FRCS
DONALD S. GARBUZ, MD, FRCSC
CLIVE P. DUNCAN, MB, MSc, FRCSC

Now that the techniques for joint replacements have been perfected, we have entered the era of increased efficiency and rapid rehabilitation. Whereas many surgical techniques have been replaced by more minimally invasive techniques, major parts of orthopaedics have lagged behind, including joint arthroplasty.

Minimally invasive hip arthroplasty was introduced to the orthopaedic community several years ago with much fanfare. This led orthopaedic surgeons to critically examine the length of the incision and the extent of deep dissection that is required to consistently result in a safe and durable outcome. The premise was that minimally invasive surgery reduces morbidity, reduces pain, shortens the length of stay, and improves overall patient satisfaction.

Furthermore, with the increasing demand on resources, such techniques could potentially allow surgeons to do more for less, by allowing patients to leave the hospital sooner. Patient demand is also a driving force and as a consequence, the minimally invasive approach is here to stay. The purpose of this article is to discuss one of these techniques, namely, the limited incision direct lateral transmuscular approach (L-TM) for total hip arthroplasty (THA).[1]

## SELECTION OF PATIENTS

For minimally invasive THA to be acceptable, it must be a predictable operation in the hands of orthopaedic surgeons who perform limited numbers of total hip arthroplasties. The direct lateral approach provides access to the hip joint through the anterior hip capsule directly through the abductors. This transgluteal approach was first described by Bauer and associates[2] in 1979 and popularized in 1982 by Hardinge[3] based on the concept of the McFarland and Osborne[4] approach which took advantage of the gluteus medius and vastus lateralis being in functional continuity through the thick periosteum covering the greater trochanter. The direct lateral is an approach that many surgeons have been trained on and are familiar with and allows preservation of the posterior soft-tissue envelope. For the minimally invasive or limited incision direct lateral approach, no special techniques or specific instruments are required, and little additional training is needed.

## Inclusion/Exclusion Criteria

With experience, all patients are possible candidates for hip arthroplasty using this approach. On the initial learning curve with this technique, patients with low body mass index and a mobile hip joint are ideal candidates. Once a surgeon is familiar with all the nuances of the technique, it can be extended to patients who have a more difficult body habitus and those with dysplasia, posttraumatic arthritis, and protrusio acetabuli.

Patients who underwent previous surgery around the hip in childhood, with scarring or instrumentation in situ, or with severe dysplasia with associated limb-length discrepancies are contraindications to performing limited incision hip arthroplasty. These patients tend to have distorted femoral anatomy and we feel that without adequate exposure, component malposition and the risk of complications will be unnecessarily high.

## SURGICAL TECHNIQUE

### Preoperative Planning

Appropriate radiographs of the pelvis and a lateral view of the hip are obtained to allow preoperative templating. The specific objectives of preoperative planning include calculation of any limb-length discrepancy and appropriate femoral offset and determination of component sizes. Limb-length discrepancies need to be corrected and femoral offset restored. At the templating stage, three important measurements are taken to aid intraoperative decision making for the femoral osteotomy and the seating of the components (**Figure 1**). The first measurement is the distance from the saddle of the neck to where the definitive osteotomy is to be performed. The second measurement is the distance from the lesser trochanter to the point of the femoral osteotomy. The last measurement is from the tip of the greater trochanter to the shoulder of the prosthesis when seating the final component. These measurements allow precise placement of components with minimal error.

The skin incision differs from the classic lateral approach as described by Bauer and associates[2] or

FIGURE 1

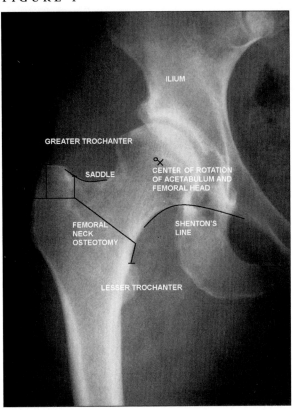

Radiograph of the right hip demonstrating the three measurements used for templating to help aid component placement: (1) the distance from the saddle to the femoral neck osteotomy; (2) the distance from the lesser trochanter to the medial femoral neck osteotomy; and (3) the distance from the tip of the greater trochanter to the shoulder of the prosthesis.

Hardinge[3] (**Figure 2**). The principle is to create a mobile window that is optimally placed for preparation of the acetabulum and the femur, and for insertion of both components. Although the mobile window concept is important, the key is still precise placement of the skin incision. This approach allows for the insertion of both cemented and cementless prosthetic components. Preoperatively all patients receive a prophylactic dose of a third-generation cephalosporin if not allergic. Most patients are given a spinal anesthetic.

The patient is positioned in the lateral decubitus position and the pelvis is supported by a pelvis-stabilizing device in a predictable position ensuring the correct acetabular orientation. Only one assistant is required.

**FIGURE 2**

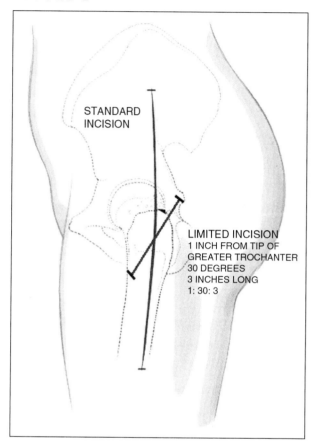

STANDARD
INCISION

LIMITED INCISION
1 INCH FROM TIP OF
GREATER TROCHANTER
30 DEGREES
3 INCHES LONG
1: 30: 3

Diagram of the standard direct lateral incision and the modification for the limited incision direct lateral approach.

The patient undergoes routine preparation and exclusion draping. The borders of the greater trochanter are palpated and marked. The skin incision is centered on a point 1 inch distal to the tip of the greater trochanter. The incision is marked 1.5 to 2 inches either side of this point (total length 3 to 4 inches), angled at 30° to the long axis of the femur with the proximal end positioned posterior-superiorly and the distal limb anteroinferiorly (**Figure 2**). The surface markings are easily remembered using the 1: 30: 3 rule, ie, 1 inch from the tip of the greater trochanter, 30° to the long axis of the femur, and 3 inches in length. The fat is cut in line with the skin using cautery to help maintain hemostasis. Soft tissue is dissected off the fascia so that the skin can move independent of the fascia. The fascial incision is made in line

with the long axis of the femur and extended 1 to 2 cm proximal and distal to the skin incision.

The plane between the tensor fascia lata and the gluteus medius is developed by blunt dissection. The leg is placed on a Mayo table to help develop this plane. A self-retaining retractor is placed underneath the fascia lata. The vastus lateralis and gluteus medius are now exposed. The junction of the anterior and posterior half of gluteus medius is identified and the fibers are separated in line to reveal adipose tissue superficial to the gluteus minimus. This fat is swept off the gluteus minimus and two retractors are placed to maintain this exposure (**Figure 3**). The fibers of the gluteus minimus are at an orientation of at least 60° more vertical than the line of the gluteus medius fibers. This finding should be recognized so as not to inadvertently divide the minimus tendon. The gluteal split should not extend more than 4 cm proximal to the greater trochanter to avoid damaging the superior gluteal neurovascular bundle. The gluteus minimus is incised along the line of its fibers and then distally this incision is curved laterally to exit in line with the incision in the gluteus medius. The extent of the distal incision is marked out and an oscillating saw is used to elevate a sliver of bone from the greater trochanter, mobilizing the composite flap of the gluteus medius, minimus, and fibers of the vasti in continuity. The sliver of bone should be no more than 2 cm long and wide and 2 mm thick (**Figure 4**). The flake of bone is grasped and dissection using cautery is continued, releasing the remainder of the gluteus minimus from the greater trochanter. The minimus is adherent to the underlying capsule and a plane is developed to the superior aspect of the acetabulum, avoiding inadvertent entry into the joint. Distally, fibers of the vastus lateralis are elevated off the capsule to optimize exposure. To aid development of this plane, the leg is slightly flexed, adducted, and gradually externally rotated. Once a clear plane between muscle and the capsule has been achieved, a narrow cobra retractor is placed around the anterior column and a smooth Steinmann pin is passed superior to the acetabulum into the ilium to help retract the abductor musculature. Alternatively, a Charnley retractor can be used to retract the composite flap. A full anterior capsulectomy is performed to expose the femoral head. The inferior capsule is released to allow the surgeon to admit one finger. After an adequate capsulectomy, the Steinmann pins are removed and the hip

**FIGURE 3**

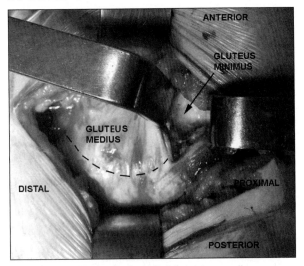

The anterior half and posterior half of the gluteus medius are separated along the line of the fibers, being careful not to extend more than 4 cm proximal to the greater trochanter. The fat covering the underlying gluteus minimus is easily seen.

**FIGURE 4**

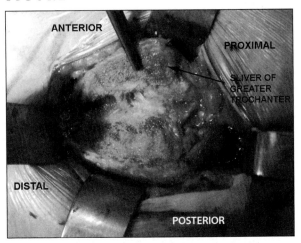

Intraoperative photograph showing elevated bone sliver from the greater trochanter.

is dislocated using a controlled maneuver involving traction, 40° to 50° of flexion, adduction, and external rotation, and the foot is placed in a sterile drape pocket on the anterior side of the table. A broad spoon-shaped elevator placed superior to the femoral head can help in this step. The leg is then rotated perpendicular to the floor, and the femoral neck osteotomy is performed as per templating using the measurements described above (**Figure 5**).

As an alternate approach, the plane of dissection can be deep to the capsule, elevating the glutei and capsule as one composite flap. Attention is then turned to the acetabulum, and two retractors are used to aid exposure. The first retractor is placed anterosuperiorly in the 2 o'clock position (for the right hip) below the capsule to protect the femoral neurovascular bundle with the leg slightly flexed, adducted, and externally rotated because this takes the tension off the psoas and rectus femoris. The transverse acetabular ligament is released with electrocautery and the second retractor is positioned posteroinferiorly in the ischium to help retract the femur. A superiorly placed smooth Steinmann pin can be used to help retract the superior capsule and abductor musculature. This allows visualization of the acetabulum (**Figure 6**). The floor is identified, remov-

ing any soft tissue in the base and a complete labrectomy is performed. Sequential reamers are used to remove eburnated bone so that bleeding bone is exposed. The acetabulum is deepened to the level as required from preoperative planning to maintain normal offset and obtain adequate lateral cup coverage. Standard reamers usually suffice, but if the patient has a large body habitus there is a tendency for the soft tissues to impinge on the handle leading to excessive reaming of the dome and a vertically malpositioned cup. Therefore, in these situations, an offset reamer can avoid this problem and malpositioned components. Reaming is carried out until rim contact is achieved with a 40° to 45° lateral opening and a 15° to 20° anterior opening (anteversion). When impacting the definitive component, an offset impactor is used to avoid impingement on the anterior soft tissues that would otherwise coax the socket into excessive lateral and/or excessive anterior opening (**Figure 7**). This inscotor has a solid force transmission unit and has an alignment jig that will guide the surgeon as to the correct lateral and anterior composite orientation of the socket.

If a cementless acetabular shell is used, screws can be inserted using a standard technique. We drill the entry point and put in a standard 30-mm screw because anything larger is difficult to insert with the correct trajectory. Any excess soft tissue that may cause impingement is removed, as are osteophytes. The liner is inserted and

**FIGURE 5**

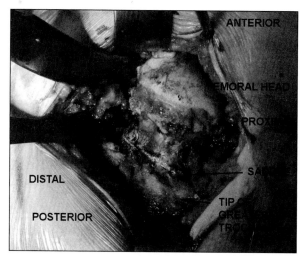

Intraoperative photograph showing the femoral head and neck and the site of the proposed osteotomy.

**FIGURE 6**

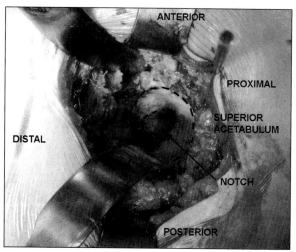

Intraoperative photograph showing the exposed acetabulum.

all retractors are removed. An elevated rim liner is seldom required if the shell orientation is correct, because of the inherent stability of this soft-tissue approach.

Attention is then turned to the femur. The leg is flexed, adducted, and externally rotated and placed in the leg bag. A femoral neck elevator can be used in larger patients to deliver the femur into the wound (**Figure 8**). A standard technique is used to prepare the femur, specific to the implant system favored by the surgeon. An assessment of whether the trochanter is over the medullary canal is made from preoperative radiographs (trochanter over medulla—TOM sign) to determine how much lateralization is required to avoid varus placement of the femoral stem.

At this point, leg length is confirmed with two measurements: the distance from the lesser trochanter to the medial extent of the femoral neck osteotomy and a suitable point on the component; as well as the distance from the tip of the greater trochanter down to the shoulder of the component. If favored by the surgeon, any one of a number of jig systems can be used to measure leg length from a fixed point on the pelvis to a mark on the greater trochanter. This is not routinely used at our institution.

Both cemented and cementless prosthetic designs can be used with this approach. Appropriate trials are carried out to assess stability of the components in all at-

risk positions, looking for possible impingement zones, soft-tissue tension, leg lengths, and lastly range of motion. The femoral component is implanted and the femoral head trial is performed again, followed by use of the definitive component. Thorough lavage with saline containing neomycin sulfate is used for irrigation. The hip is relocated.

The composite flap of the gluteus medius, vastus lateralis, and gluteus minimus are reduced to their anatomic position and securely repaired to the femur using tendon-to-tendon or bone flap-to-bone repair. The flake of bone can be used as a guide to the correct position of the flap, allowing appropriate tensioning. We favor the use of a nonabsorbable braided suture passed through drill holes in the greater trochanter and around the flake of bone in the substance of the gluteal tendon (**Figure 9**). The fascia lata, fat, and skin then are closed in separate layers. We favor the infiltration of local anesthetic after wound closure to facilitate postoperative pain management.

## PITFALLS AND COMMON ERRORS

Limited incision total hip arthroplasty has its own set of pitfalls and common errors, including the following: (1) If struggling to gain exposure, have a low threshold to extend the incision, especially in the learning phase.

FIGURE 7

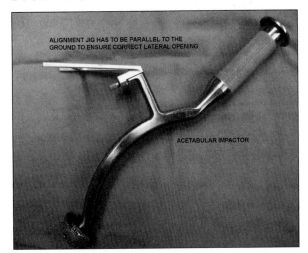

Limited incision acetabular impactor.

FIGURE 8

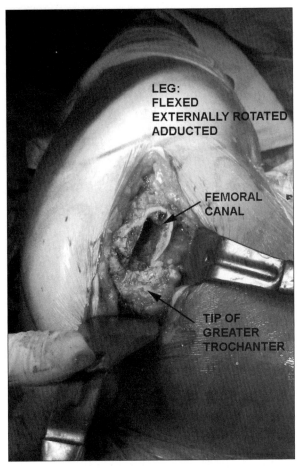

Exposure of the femoral canal.

(2) It is advisable to raise at least 50% of the anterior abductors as a composite flap to avoid damage to the remaining abductors. (3) If taking a sliver of bone with the abductors, do not take too thick or thin a slice. If too thick, there is a chance of subsequent fracture of the greater trochanter. If too thin, the sliver can fragment. (4) At no point should the dissection in the gluteus medius and minimus extend beyond 4 cm proximal to the greater trochanter, so as to preserve the superior gluteal neurovascular bundle. (5) With increasing experience, a T-shaped capsulotomy as opposed to a capsulectomy can be performed, allowing later repair. However, we feel that the approach is inherently stable and that this is not required; but in the presence of atrophied abductors, this may add to the stability. (6) Avoid cutting the neck long because visualization of the acetabulum is difficult and subsequent recutting is required. In the limited incision technique, if there is capsular tightness, the neck cut can be intentionally low to decrease tension and provide more mobility to the deeper tissues, with appropriate adjustment of the femoral component and upsizing if deemed appropriate to ensure no limb-length discrepancy. (7) In larger patients, consider using an offset reamer to avoid deflection by the soft tissues and malposition of the cup. If there is a rim osteophyte, this should be removed to allow better visualization and ease of placement of reamers. (8) Be aware if using offset reamers to appreciate the orientation of alignment jigs to achieve correct lateral opening and version position. (9) We prefer to use full hemisphere reamers. For those using "cut-off" reamers, be careful to avoid jumping and eccentric reaming. It is helpful to have the reamer rotating before engaging the acetabulum. When reaming, choose a reamer that is close to the final reamer to be used to avoid creating two concavities. (10) Use a standard rim liner except in special cases, as reduction can be difficult. Because this approach is inherently stable, it avoids the need for offset or oblique face liners. (11) If it is difficult to deliver the femur, even with a femoral elevator, then a release involving the posteromedial tissues without inadvertent release of the psoas should allow further mobilization

FIGURE 9

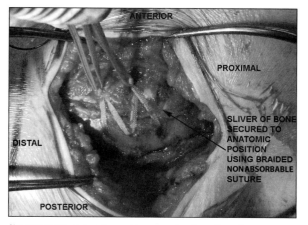

Nonabsorbable suture is used to secure the bony flap closure.

and aid delivery. (12) When approaching the femur for canal preparation, the use of femoral elevators and longitudinal pressure to the knee help deliver the femur into the proximal aspect of the incision. When broaching the femur, the proximal skin edge can be traumatized; therefore, at this stage the surgeon should have a low threshold to extend the incision 0.5 to 1 cm to avoid this. (13) If the broach is smaller than expected and there is difficulty advancing it, it is likely that it is malaligned into varus. Confirm that the appropriate degree of lateralization has been achieved and ensure that a trough has been created in the medial face of the greater trochanter. Then advance the broaches again. (14) When securing the bone fragment or the musculotendinous composite flap, always tie the knots anterior to avoid soft-tissue irritation and trochanteric bursitis.

## POSTOPERATIVE REGIMEN

The postoperative regimen follows the standard protocol including prophylactic antibiotics administered for 24 hours and low-molecular-weight heparin for 10 days. More extended prophylaxis is required for those at greater risk of developing a thromboembolism. A multimodal management strategy for pain, nausea, and blood loss has been devised in conjunction with the orthopaedic surgeons and anesthesiologists. This is commenced before surgery.

All patients undergo a standardized program of accel-erated rehabilitation, starting with mobilization on the same day as surgery. Activities are encouraged simultaneously and not on a step-by-step basis. All activities are supervised and if a patient attains the criteria set, they are discharged when deemed safe. Immediate weight bearing is encouraged, but active abduction is discouraged for 6 weeks to allow the bone fragment and attached glutei to heal. Patients are typically discharged home on day 3, after reaching the expected rehabilitation milestones.

## OUR EXPERIENCE

### Results

Previously our unit has reported on a prospective cohort of 50 patients undergoing this limited incision direct lateral approach for total hip arthroplasty and compared them to a cohort of 56 patients undergoing a standard approach, defining differences in the duration of the surgery, the type of prosthesis used, blood loss, percentage of hemoglobin deficits, transfusion requirements, length of stay, and complications.[5] Demographically, the body mass index (BMI) was significantly lower in the limited incision group ($P < 0.007$), and there was a greater preponderance of male patients in this subgroup. There was no difference in other baseline parameters including age or comorbidities. The ratio of cementless to hybrid total hip arthroplasties in the limited incision group was 2.6 and 1.6 in the control group. Significant differences were noted in the duration of operations with limited incision hip arthroplasties taking 13 minutes longer on average, 82-mL less estimated blood loss, and a reduced length of stay by 1.3 days compared to the standard group. Transfusion requirements were no different. Complications were minimal in both groups, with two stable intraoperative fractures in the limited incision group treated by cerclage wiring. In the limited incision group, the following were encountered: one patient with a thigh hematoma, one patient with bowel pseudo-obstruction that resolved, one patient with pseudomembranous colitis, and one patient with a ventricular tachycardia that spontaneously reverted. In the control group, one patient had postoperative confusion and another was diagnosed with neurocardiogenic syncope. There was an obvious selection bias for those undergoing limited incision hip arthroplasty which would have influenced the results, but this is expected in the surgeons' initial learning curve.

More recently we have prospectively reviewed a cohort of 68 patients undergoing the limited incision direct lateral approach and 115 patients undergoing a standard direct lateral approach for total hip arthroplasty and have assessed patient-based quality of life scores using the WOMAC index, satisfaction scores, and radiologic parameters at 1-year follow-up. The distribution of diagnoses was similar in both groups, with primary osteoarthritis being the major category. There was no significant difference in age/sex distribution or comorbidities. BMI was significantly different, with limited incision patients having lower BMIs. When comparing quality of life scores, satisfaction scores, and radiographic positioning, there was no statistically significant difference between groups. Complications were similar in both groups.

## THE LITERATURE

There have been few studies comparing the limited incision direct lateral approach to other approaches for primary total hip arthroplasty. There are no randomized controlled trials. There are several studies, two of which are a consecutive series of case-controlled patients including ours, and one is a matched cohort study. Our experience has been described.

deBeer and associates[6] reported that in 30 limited incision and 30 standard cases that the only measurable advantage was a reduced blood loss of 67 mL; there were no differences in requirements of blood transfusion, length of stay, incidence of complications, or component malpositioning. They advocated that the length of the skin incision is clinically and functionally irrelevant.

O'Brien and Rorabeck[7] reviewed 34 total hip arthroplasties done using a mini-incision direct lateral approach with 53 patients undergoing the standard approach. They demonstrated that the advantage of limited incision hip arthroplasty was a 6-minute reduced surgical time that was probably not clinically significant and a 1-day reduction in length of stay. Radiographically the mean abduction angle was 45° for both groups. The femoral stem alignment was within 5° of neutral in 97% of the mini group and 94% of the standard group. There were no dislocations, infections, or neurologic or wound

complications. The intraoperative fracture rate in the limited incision group was 6%, and it was 2% in the standard group ($P > 0.05$). They also demonstrated a selection bias in regards to BMI when considering groups, and concluded that it was safe to continue further study in the form of a randomized controlled study with this limited incision direct lateral approach because there was no increase in complications or component malpositioning.

## DISCUSSION

The clinical studies to date with limited incision surgery using a single direct lateral incision have demonstrated that this operation is safe and effective and although there are no major advantages, the outcomes are no worse when considering factors such as complications or component orientation. There may be decreased surgical time, decreased length of hospital stay, and improved discharge dispositions with the mini-incision approach, but long-term benefits in terms of function and pain have not been documented in the literature.

Our data support the concept that there are significant improvements in quality of life scores in this group undergoing primary THA and that there is no statistically significant difference when comparing scores to the standard approach. Therefore, this approach does not have a negative impact on outcomes at 1-year follow-up. However, it is difficult to draw definite conclusions from our data because of selection bias and the fact that it is a consecutive series. The only way to avoid this is to set up a randomized controlled study. Radiographic outcome revealed minimal outliers and high satisfaction scores in this group of patients. Our results show that this is a reproducible technique with no adverse effects and its continued use is justified.

Cosmesis is another important implication for patients, especially those who require hip arthroplasty at a younger age. Patients do want minimally invasive operations to be safe and effective and this is borne out in the literature for all types of minimally invasive approaches.[8-11] If the same component position can be reliably achieved, then there is no reason to suspect inferior outcomes and decreased longevity of implants. Anecdotally, most patients are impressed by smaller incisions. They equate smaller incisions with efficiency and improved outcomes. If a surgeon can perform the operation in a manner that increases the psychological well-being of the patient, then he or she should be motivated to use such a method for the benefit of the patient. As the surgeon's experience expands, then adverse outcomes are minimized and reproducibility and quality maintained.

This limited incision direct lateral approach is a variation on a traditional approach that is familiar to all orthopaedic surgeons. Limited training is required, with minimal specialized techniques involved and the use of standard equipment. It provides excellent visualization, is easy to use, requires only one assistant, and for those who use a standard direct lateral approach and have the experience, it is an easy modification to make, with little change in operating room practices and without compromise of component positioning.

As with all limited incision techniques, further research into various aspects of this technology need to be addressed, including long-term durability of the joint reconstruction, long-term outcome of pain and function parameters, implant orientation, infection rates, incidence and prevalence of deep venous thrombosis, and other complications including neurovascular injury, dislocation, and revision rate. Factors such as safety, efficacy, and cost effectiveness should also be evaluated before widespread dissemination of this technique.

## REFERENCES

1. Duncan CP, Toms A, Masri BA: Minimally invasive or limited incision hip replacement: Clarification and classification. *Instr Course Lect* 2006;55:195-197.
2. Bauer R, Kerschbaumer F, Poisel S, Oberthaler W: The transgluteal approach to the hip joint. *Arch Orthop Trauma Surg* 1979;95:47-49.
3. Hardinge K: The direct lateral approach to the hip. *J Bone Joint Surg Br* 1982;64:17-19.
4. McFarland B, Osborne G: Approach to the hip: A suggested improvement on use of braided Kocher's method. *J Bone Joint Surg Br* 1954;36:364-367.
5. Howell JR, Masri BA, Duncan CP: Minimally invasive versus standard incision anterolateral hip replacement: A comparative study. *Orthop Clin North Am* 2004;35:153-162.
6. deBeer J, Petruccelli D, Zalzal P, et al: Single-incision, minimally invasive total hip arthroplasty: Length doesn't matter. *J Arthroplasty* 2004;19:945.
7. O'Brien DA, Rorabeck CH: The mini-incision direct lateral approach in primary total hip arthroplasty. *Clin Orthop Relat Res* 2005;441:99-103.
8. Ogonda L, Wilson R, Archbold P, et al: Minimal-incision technique in THA does not improve early postoperative outcomes: A prospective randomized controlled trial. *J Bone Joint Surg Am* 2005;87:701-710.
9. Wright JM, Crockett HC, Delgado S, et al: Mini-incision for total hip arthroplasty: A prospective, controlled, investigation with 5 year follow-up evaluation. *J Arthroplasty* 2004;19:538-545.
10. Wenz JF, Gurkan I, Jibodh SR: Mini-incision total hip arthroplasty: A comparative assessment of perioperative outcomes. *Orthopedics* 2002;25:1031-1043.
11. DiGioia A, Plakseychuck A, Levison T, et al: Mini-incision technique for total hip arthroplasty with navigation. *J Arthroplasty* 2003;18:123-128.

# CHAPTER 5

# LIMITED INCISION POSTERIOR APPROACH FOR TOTAL HIP ARTHROPLASTY

JEFFREY L. BUSH, MD
THOMAS PARKER VAIL, MD

For decades, the posterior approach to the hip[1,2] has provided excellent functional results. It allows safe access to the hip joint while sparing the abductor attachments, thus causing a low incidence of postoperative abductor weakness and abnormal gait. The direct lateral[3] and modified lateral approaches have been associated with an incidence of postoperative abductor weakness and slower recovery due to the need to protect the abductor mechanism repair.[4] A negative aspect of the posterior approach has been a slightly higher rate of dislocation, especially when using smaller diameter femoral head prostheses.[5,6] Improvements in bearing surfaces leading to increased clinical use of larger diameter bearings, as well as the recognition of the importance of anatomic posterior capsular repair, have lowered the dislocation rate and enabled the posterior approach to become a very stable approach to hip arthroplasty.[7-9] The minimally invasive posterior approach is an evolution of this standard posterior approach.

Although it has become ubiquitous in the field of orthopaedics, the term "minimally invasive surgery" does not have a true definition. The terminology certainly implies that an incision smaller than the standard incisions of the past will be used. Ideally, minimally inva-sive surgery involves the elimination of all parts of the standard incision that are not necessary to successfully complete the operation, making the terminology "limited incision surgery" perhaps more accurate. The smaller incision can be considered a "mobile window" through which the procedure is done, allowing visualization of different anatomic structures as the procedure unfolds. It should be considered an extensile approach that can be lengthened as needed during a given surgery. The necessary incision length may become smaller as the comfort level of the surgeon increases.

The limited incision posterior approach to the hip uses a small portion of the standard posterior approach to the hip, passing through the same muscular and nervous intervals. Modifications in techniques and instrumentation have allowed safe access to the hip through a smaller incision.[10-14] Minimizing the length of the skin incision, however, should not be the goal of surgery. The ideal length of incision is the smallest required to safely perform the operation. Generally, this can be done with an incision of 8 to 15 cm (3 to 6 inches). The length is determined by the size of the patient and the depth of the acetabulum within the soft tissues. A larger or more muscular patient will require a longer incision.

## PATIENT SELECTION

Any primary hip replacement can be done using the limited incision posterior approach with the technique discussed in this chapter. The important point for patients and surgeons alike to consider is the fact that the length of the incision will vary from patient to patient depending on the amount of fat, the degree of muscularity, and the compliance of the tissues. Thus, the limited incision selection criteria is not "one size fits all," but rather a technique that can be applied and adapted in all cases. Specific contraindications would be those complicated cases of hip replacement after prior surgery necessitating the need for an extended exposure to remove retained hardware, expose the sciatic nerve, perform an osteotomy, and the majority of revision cases.

## PREOPERATIVE PATIENT EDUCATION

Although rarely mentioned in the literature, preoperative patient education is an important aspect of minimal incision hip surgery. With easy access to information via the Internet, and widespread marketing at all levels from device companies to individual practice, patients are at risk of developing unrealistic expectations about their hip replacement procedure. It is important for surgeons to define for their patients exactly what is meant by minimally invasive surgery in their practice. Patients should also understand that it is not only the surgical technique, but also the anesthesia, pain management, and rehabilitation protocols that facilitate a rapid recovery from hip surgery.

## SURGICAL TECHNIQUE

The procedure is performed with the patient in the lateral decubitus position. All pressure points are well padded and an axillary pad is placed under the upper thorax. A pelvic positioning device is used to stabilize the pelvis during the procedure. The skin incision is a short oblique incision centered over the posterior aspect of the acetabulum[15] (**Figure 1**). It should be in line with the proposed path of acetabular reaming, which is essentially in line with the fibers of the gluteus maximus muscle. Palpable surface landmarks include the tip of the greater trochanter, the sciatic notch, and the anterior edge of the vastus lateralis ridge. The incision is placed

FIGURE 1

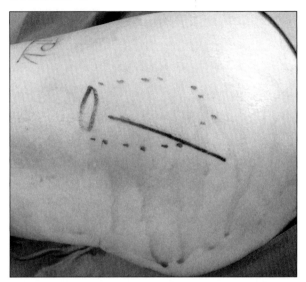

With the patient in the lateral position, the skin incision should be centered over the posterior aspect of the acetabulum and in line with the proposed path of reaming.

within the line created by connecting the sciatic notch with the posterior edge of the vastus ridge, thus paralleling the femoral shaft when the hip is flexed approximately 45°. The initial incision should measure approximately 4 to 5 cm in length and can be extended proximally or distally as needed during the procedure. Roughly one third of the incision is above the tip of the trochanter, and two thirds of the incision is below the tip. Skin stretching should be kept to a minimum during the procedure. The necessity to stretch the skin means that the incision is not long enough. To maximize visualization and minimize skin stretching or other soft-tissue trauma, the number of instruments placed in the wound at a time should be kept to a minimum and self-retaining retractors are used sparingly or not at all.

After the skin incision, sharp dissection is carried down to the level of the fascia over the gluteus maximus and tensor fascia muscles. Avoid unnecessary trauma to the fat layer, which can lead to devascularization. The fascia is divided in line with the fibers of the gluteus maximus, which are then separated bluntly to expose the posterior hip joint located just beneath the trochanteric bursal tissue. Carefully control bleeding points with electrocautery. Avoid cutting or tearing mus-

**FIGURE 2**

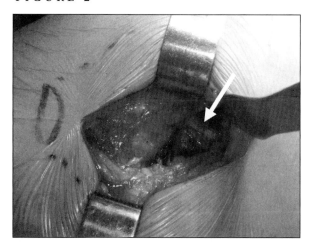

The posterior hip joint has been exposed. The piriformis tendon is visible in the proximal aspect of the incision. The hip joint is entered in the interval between the superior edge of the piriformis and the inferior edge of the gluteus minimus.

cle fibers. Distally, the fascia is divided to the level of the muscle-tendon junction of the tensor fascia muscle. A standard Charnley retractor may then be placed beneath the gluteus maximus muscle fibers and superficial to the tendon of the gluteus medius. Care should be taken to not stretch the skin or damage the muscle when placing the retractor. When using a very small incision, the Charnley retractor can place excessive tension on the skin; therefore, a smaller self-retaining retractor may be more appropriate. In addition, the surgeon should be aware that if the posterior Charnley retractor is placed too deep, the sciatic nerve may be in danger.

After separation of the gluteus maximus muscle fibers and internal rotation of the hip, the posterior aspect of the greater trochanter and trochanteric bursa are well visualized. The bursa can be divided or swept posteriorly revealing the piriformis and short external rotators (**Figure 2**). Exposure is assisted by placing a blunt homan retractor beneath the gluteus medius tendon and on top of the gluteus minumus tendon, passing around the front of the femoral neck. The posterior border of the medius is thereby gently elevated, exposing the interval between the superior edge of the piriformis and the inferior edge of the gluteus minimus. Excessive traction on the posterior edge of the gluteus medius muscle should

be avoided so as to minimize the risk of any traction on the greater sciatic neurovascular bundle which emerges from the sciatic notch.

Next, the posterior capsular incision is made to expose the hip joint. The hip capsule and short external rotators can be excised separately or together to expose the hip. The key concept with the capsular incision is to create a strong flap of capsule and tendon that can be repaired anatomically. Typically, an L-shaped capsulotomy is made, starting along the superior border of the piriformis (and the posterior edge of the gluteus minimus muscle) and proceeding distally to the piriformis fossa, then along the intertrochanteric line to the proximal edge of the quadratus femoris muscle. In most patients, the quadratus can be left intact. The proximal extent of the capsular exposure is the rim of the acetabulum. The capsulotendinous flap is tagged with suture and reflected posteriorly. Often a plexus of veins overlying the short external rotators will require cauterization as the posterior capsule and external rotators are incised. The hip is then dislocated with flexion and internal rotation. Tension on the sciatic nerve is reduced by keeping the knee flexed at all times.

The femoral neck cut is made according to the preoperative plan based on measurement down from the tip of the greater trochanter or up from the lesser trochanter. When using a small incision, it can be helpful to cut the neck in a segmental fashion, first making a subcapital cut and removing the femoral head. After making the femoral neck cut, the leg is placed back in neutral rotation with slight hip flexion and the acetabulum is exposed.

The most important aspect in acetabular exposure is the proper mobilization of the proximal femur. The hip must be flexed and the proximal femur translated anteriorly to allow sufficient room for concentric reaming of the acetabulum. A curved anterior retractor is placed under the femoral neck and over the anterior rim of the acetabulum. With this retractor in place, the anterior fibers of the hip capsule are placed under tension. These can be elevated off of the anterior column to facilitate anterior translation of the femur and adequate visualization of the acetabulum (**Figure 3**). In some patients, a tight inferior capsule tethers the anterior translation of the femur. In this instance, a radial cut can be made in the inferior capsule. The radial cut in the capsule extends perpendicular to and longitudinally outward

**FIGURE 3**

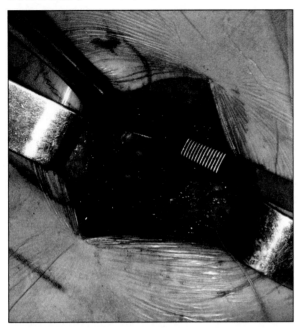

The fibers of the anterior hip capsule are sharply elevated off of the superior and anterior aspect of the acetabulum. Mobilization of the capsule allows anterior translation of the proximal femur so that the acetabulum can be properly exposed.

**FIGURE 4**

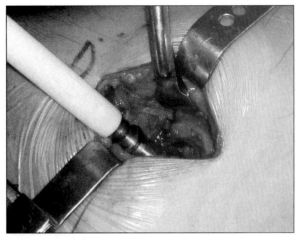

During reaming, the anterior acetabular retractor is used to translate the proximal femur anteriorly and distally so that it does not interfere with the direction of reaming. Posteriorly, the tagging sutures pull the capsule away from the reamer. Note that a minimum of instruments are placed in the wound during reaming.

from the transverse acetabular ligament. The transverse acetabular ligament may be left intact when the inferior capsule is divided as it does not constrain movement of the femur. Care should be taken to coagulate branches of the obturator artery that exit the obturator foramen adjacent to the transverse acetabular ligament. With the acetabulum now completely visualized, the labrum can be sharply excised and acetabular reaming can begin.

When reaming the acetabulum through a smaller incision, it is important to make sure the direction of reaming is not dictated by the skin edges, proximal femur, or retractors (**Figure 4**). With the hip flexed and the anterior retractor in place, the femur should be retracted away from the reamer. Posteriorly, the capsule is kept away from the reamer by pulling upward on the tagging sutures. By retracting the femur distally and anteriorly, the overlying skin moves distally with the retractors. This allows reaming in the proper acetabular orientation without placing excessive stretch on the skin. In some systems, modified, or S-shaped reamers can be used to ream in the appropriate orientation without placing

excess tension on the skin and soft tissues. A modified cup inserter can accomplish the same thing once reaming is completed.

After placement of the acetabular component, the next step is exposure of the proximal femur and preparation for the femoral component. The hip is flexed and internally rotated. A narrow proximal femoral elevator is placed under the remaining femoral neck (**Figure 5**). A sharp homan retractor is placed above the lesser trochanter, around the femoral calcar. The surgical assistant plays an important role in keeping the proximal femur centered in the incision and applying axial pressure to push the femur into the incision. Careful manipulation of the proximal femoral elevator and the leg allows better visualization of the piriformis fossa or femoral calcar at different points in the operation. This helps ensure appropriate fit of the implant and minimizes the risk of calcar or femoral fracture during the procedure. Standard preparation of the femur for a given implant system is then performed. Trial components can be placed to assess range of motion, length, stability, and points of impingement. An intraoperative radiograph can be used at this time to confirm size and position of the implants and restoration of appropriate leg length.

Next, the final femoral components are placed. Dur-

FIGURE 5

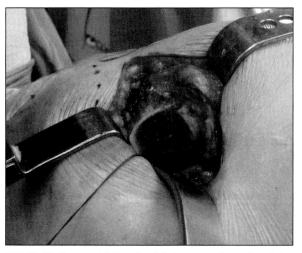

With the hip flexed and internally rotated, a narrow femoral neck elevator is used to expose the proximal femur.

ing implant insertion, it is critical to keep them from touching the skin edges. This limits potential bacterial contamination. The incision must be long enough to accommodate this process. Femoral component insertion may require movement of the femur from the flexed and internally rotated position after the tip of the implant is in the femoral canal, to a more extended position that relaxes the posterior skin edge and allows the neck and trunion of the implant to pass into the wound. Once the prosthesis is completely within the surgical wound, the hip is again flexed and internally rotated for final seating of the implant with direct visualization of the femoral calcar. Similarly, the prosthesis may need to be rotated carefully into the incision to avoid contact with the skin, ensuring the appropriate amount of anteversion once the trunion is within the incision and the calcar is clearly visible (**Figure 6**). The wound is closed in layers starting with repair of the hip capsule. The repair is done anatomically, by either pulling the piriformis tendon down toward the piriformis fossa by passing the sutures through the anterior portion of the gluteus medius tendon or through trochanteric drill holes. This repair has been shown to decrease the dislocation rate following a posterior approach to the hip, especially when using smaller head sizes.[5,6] Finally, the fascia, subcutaneous layer, and skin are closed and a sterile dressing is applied.

## PITFALLS AND COMMON ERRORS

Limited incision hip surgery is not without complications. Improper reaming of the acetabulum, vertical cup placement, intraoperative fractures, and prolonged surgical time have all been reported. In a report of three disastrous complications, Fehring and Mason[16] noted that surgeon inexperience was a contributing factor in each case.

Along with surgeon inexperience, errors in limited incision surgery are most likely the result of the difficulty encountered by working through a smaller surgical portal. The surgeon cannot allow the skin, retractors, or improper mobilization of the femur to compromise the acetabular preparation. Placing the incision in the proper location in line with the angle of reaming can facilitate this. Use of an accessory incision for placement of the reamer has also been described; a small incision is made where the surgeon would like the reamer to be positioned.[17] The reamer shaft is inserted through the accessory incision and attached to the reamer head inside the main incision.

Although the shorter incision is a significant aspect of minimally invasive hip surgery, the shorter scar is not always more appealing than the standard scars of the past. Mow and associates[18] evaluated surgical scars after standard and mini-posterior total hip approaches. Twenty mini-incision and 14 standard approaches were compared at an average of 2 years postoperatively. Blinded observers, who were practicing plastic surgeons not involved in the surgeries, found that more of the mini scars rated poorly than standard scars. When polled, all patients involved in the study rated pain relief and longevity as higher priorities than scar cosmesis, but the study did not comprehensively address the patients' satisfaction with cosmesis. This study raises the important point that stretching the skin may allow the surgeon to measure a shorter incision, but it does not always equate with a more cosmetic scar and can actually lead to increased wound complications.

## POSTOPERATIVE CARE

The interest in limited incision hip arthroplasty has coincided with an effort to adapt anesthesia and rehabilitation protocols to promote more rapid recovery from surgery. In some cases, the perceived benefit of

FIGURE 6

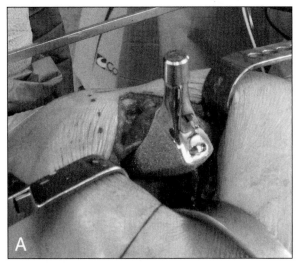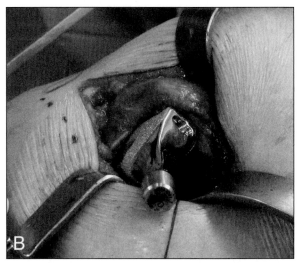

**A,** Care is taken to insert the femoral component without contacting the skin edges. The distal part of the stem can be inserted into the femoral canal with the neck and trunion pointed away from the skin edge to avoid skin contact. **B,** The stem is then rotated into the proper version once in the wound and impacted into place.

minimally invasive surgery should in part be attributed to improved anesthesia, postoperative pain control, and accelerated rehabilitation. Regional anesthesia protocols, including spinal and epidural anesthesia, continuous lumbar plexus blocks, and continuous peripheral nerve blocks, are currently being used to promote faster recovery from hip arthroplasty.[19] Sharkey[20] reported that with enhanced anesthesia and rehabilitation protocols, patients had earlier functional improvement, shorter time to discharge home, and increased satisfaction regardless of the length of the skin incision.

## RESULTS

Reports of limited posterior incision total hip arthroplasty vary from optimistic to negative, with most reports showing little difference in outcome directly attributable to the length of the incision. Among the more optimistic reports is that of Inaba and associates.[21] They concluded that, with experience, limited incision posterior hip arthroplasty can improve outcomes. They compared a group of 100 consecutive limited incision posterior hip arthroplasties done between 2001 and 2002 to a second group of 100 consecutive limited incision posterior hips done in 2004. With the combination of

technical and patient care improvements, they were able to obtain shorter hospital stays, less opioid use, and faster muscle recovery in the second group. These results demonstrate the value of experience with limited incision surgery, as well as the positive impact of improvements in perioperative care. Goldstein and associates[22] retrospectively reviewed 170 total hip arthroplasties, half of which were performed through a minimal posterior incision (average 13 cm) and the other half through a standard posterior incision (average 36 cm). In the smaller incision group, the authors had a lower estimated blood loss, but there was no difference in transfusion rates between the two groups. There were also no differences between the groups in surgical times or Harris hip scores preoperatively and 12 weeks postoperatively. For obese patients (BMI > 27), the results did not differ between the minimal and standard incisions.

Wright and associates[23] compared 42 small posterior surgical incisions (average 8.8 cm) to 43 standard incisions (average 23 cm). The BMI of the small incision group was significantly lower than the standard incision group (24 versus 28). The small incision group had shorter surgical times but no other advantages other than cosmetic appeal. At 5 years, Harris hip scores were equivalent and there had been no revisions in either group. In a separate study, Chimento and associates[24] prospectively compared 28 primary total hip arthroplasties randomized to small posterior incisions (8 cm) to 32 cases with larger posterior incisions (15 cm). All patients had a BMI below 30. Patients in the small incision group had significantly less estimated intraoperative blood loss and a lower rate of limp at 6 weeks, which normalized by 1 year. Surgical time, rate of transfusion, length of hospital stay, and complication rates were similar between the groups.

Wenz and associates[17] compared a retrospective series of 124 total hip arthroplasties done through a limited posterior incision (average incision 8 cm) to a series of 65 standard incision direct lateral cases (incisions ≥ 25 cm). The BMI was significantly lower in the limited posterior incision group. The limited incision group had shorter surgical times and a lower rate of blood transfusion. The limited incision patients were able to ambulate significantly sooner postoperatively, with three times the number of patients able to ambulate independently on postoperative day one compared to the standard lateral incision group. There were no significant differences in complication rates or component positioning between the two groups. Although this study compared not just incision length but also surgical approach, the limited posterior approach was found to be as safe and effective as an accepted traditional technique.

In a randomized, prospectively controlled trial of 219 hips, Ogonda and associates[25] found that limited posterior incision total hip arthroplasty was safe and reproducible but did not improve early outcomes compared to standard incisions. Patients were randomized to a short incision of ≤ 10 cm or a standard incision of 16 cm. The anesthesia, pain management, and postoperative rehabilitation protocols were the same in both groups. There were no differences between the two groups in component placement, early walking ability, or functional outcome at 6 weeks. Earlier discharge was correlated with patient age and the level of the preoperative hematocrit for both small and large incisions. Patients with a BMI above 35 had longer surgical times regardless of the incision length.

The largest published case series on a limited incision posterior approach reviewed 1,000 consecutive primary total hip arthroplasties in 759 patients who were followed for a minimum of 2 years.[26] All patients received a tapered, cementless femoral component and a press-fit acetabular shell. The mean incision length was 8.8 cm (range 6 to 16 cm). No patients were excluded on the basis of BMI (range 14.3 to 56.5). Radiographically, implant position was acceptable in 95% of cases. There were six radiographic acetabular failures in the study and no cases of femoral loosening. Complications included a dislocation rate of 3%, a deep infection rate of 0.3%, and an overall revision rate of 2.1%.

In a study that highlights the concern over the danger involved in limited incision hip arthroplasty, Woolson and associates[27] found a higher overall complication rate that did not reach statistical significance for a limited incision posterior approach than the standard posterior approach in a consecutive series of 135 patients. Nevertheless, the limited incision posterior approach was associated with a statistically significant higher risk of wound complications (6% limited incision versus 0% standard, $P = 0.02$) when the two dialysis patients that happened to be in the standard group were excluded. More concerning was the fact that in the limited incision group there were more acetabular components placed outside the target 30° to 50° abduction range (30% versus 15%, $P = 0.04$), and more femoral components with either poor fit and fill or varus position in the limited incision group (14% versus 4%, $P = 0.02$). Due to the selection process in the study, the limited incision group actually had a lower mean BMI than the standard incision group, indicating that the higher complication rate in the small incision group was not related to patient size, but to the difficulty in working through the smaller incision.

Unrecognized soft-tissue damage is another concern in limited incision hip surgery that has been part of the debate in the literature about the benefits (and potential hazards) of two-incision minimally invasive hip arthroplasty.[28] The two-incision minimally invasive approach has been proposed as a muscle-sparing approach, as compared to the posterior approach, in which the gluteus maximus is split in line with its fibers and the piriformis and short external rotators are detached from the proximal femur. Mardones and associates[29] evaluated the muscle damage created by both two-incision and mini-posterior techniques in a cadaver study. Twenty hips were studied. Muscle damage was assessed in each cadaver after a two-incision hip was performed on one hip and a mini-posterior hip on the contralateral hip. Damage to the gluteus medius and minimus muscles was substantially greater for the two-incision group than the mini-posterior group. There was no difference in the damage to the gluteal tendons between the two groups. This study refutes the notion that two-incision hip arthroplasty is muscle sparing and underscores the need for visualization and protection of soft tissues while performing limited incision hip surgery, regardless of the approach.

Computer navigation might be used to obtain proper component orientation without visualizing the usual anatomic landmarks, thus requiring less dissection and potentially expanding the role of limited incision surgery. Further experience with computer navigation will be required to prove this hypothesis. Wixson and MacDonald[30] compared 82 navigated total hips done with a minimal posterior incision to a retrospective cohort of 50 standard posterior approach hips. They found significantly more consistent acetabular component placement in the computer-navigated mini-incision group than in the standard incision group. On radiographic measurements, the navigation group had less variance in both cup abduction and flexion. Issues such as accurate registration of anatomic landmarks, need for preoperative imaging, and increased expense have yet to be fully addressed.

## Conclusions

The standard posterior approach total hip arthroplasty can evolve into a limited incision, tissue-sparing procedure with high expectations for both rapid recovery and long-term function with proper patient selection and application of the technique. However, limited incision surgery is not without risks and has a documented learning curve, even for experienced surgeons. As limited incision techniques are applied, the goal is to cultivate the use of smaller incisions combined with minimal soft-tissue damage, optimal component position, and not jeopardize patient outcome simply to make a smaller skin incision.

## References

1. Harris WH: A new approach to total hip replacement without osteotomy of the greater trochanter. *Clin Orthop Relat Res* 1975;106:19-26.
2. Moore AT: The Moore self locking vitalium prosthesis in fresh femoral neck fractures: A new low posterior approach (The Southern Exposure). *Instr Course Lect* 1959;16:309-321.
3. Hardinge K: The direct lateral approach to the hip. *J Bone Joint Surg Br* 1982;64:17-24.
4. Roberts JM, Fu FH, McCain EF, Ferguson AB: A comparison of posterolateral and anterolateral approaches to total hip arthroplasty. *Clin Orthop Relat Res* 1984;187:205.
5. Lu-Yao GL, Keller RB, Littenberg B, Wennberg JE: Outcomes after displaced fractures of the femoral neck: A meta-analysis of one hundred and six published reports. *J Bone Joint Surg Am* 1994;76:15-25.
6. Woolson ST, Rahimtoola ZO: Risk factors for dislocation during the first 3 months after primary total hip replacement. *J Arthroplasty* 1999;14:662-668.
7. Pellicci PM, Bostrom M, Poss R: Posterior approach to total hip replacement using enhanced posterior soft tissue repair. *Clin Orthop Relat Res* 1998;355:224-228.
8. Weeden SH, Paprosky WG, Bowling JW: The early dislocation rate in primary total hip arthroplasty following the posterior approach with posterior soft-tissue repair. *J Arthroplasty* 2003;18:709-713.
9. Kelley SS, Lachiewicz PF, Hickman JM, Paterno SM: Relationship of femoral head and acetabular size to the prevalence of dislocation. *Clin Orthop Relat Res* 1998;355:163-170.
10. Berry D, Berger R, Callaghan J, et al: Minimally invasive total hip arthroplasty: Development, early results and a critical analysis. *J Bone Joint Surg Am* 2003;85:2235-2246.
11. Goldstein W, Branson J: Posterior-lateral approach to minimal incision total hip arthroplasty. *Orthop Clin North Am* 2004;35:131-136.
12. Hartzband M: Posterolateral minimal incision for total hip replacement: Technique and early results. *Orthop Clin North Am* 2004;35:119-129.
13. Howell J, Garbuz D, Duncan C: Minimally invasive hip replacement: Rationale, applied anatomy, and instrumentation. *Orthop Clin North Am* 2004;35:107-118.
14. Sculco T, Jordan L, Walter W: Minimally invasive total hip arthroplasty: The Hospital for Special Surgery experience. *Orthop Clin North Am* 2004;35:137-142.
15. Vail TP: Minimal incision hip arthroplasty: The posterior mini-incision. *Semin Arthroplasty* 2004;15:83-86.
16. Fehring T, Mason J: Catastrophic complications of minimally invasive hip surgery. *J Bone Joint Surg Am* 2005;87:711-714.

17. Wenz JF, Gurkan I, Jibodh SR: Mini-incision total hip arthroplasty: A comparative assessment of perioperative outcomes. *Orthopedics* 2002;25:1031-1043.

18. Mow CS, Woolson ST, Ngarmukos SG, Park EH, Lorenz HP: Comparison of scars from total hip replacements done through standard or a mini-incision. *Clin Orthop Relat Res* 2005;441:80-85.

19. Indelli PF, Grant SA, Nielsen K, Vail TP: Regional anesthesia in hip surgery. *Clin Orthop Relat Res* 2005;441:250-255.

20. Sharkey P: Minimally invasive hip arthroplasty: What role does patient preconditioning play? Closed meeting of the Hip Society, 2005.

21. Inaba Y, Dorr LD, Wan Z, Sirianni L, Boutary M: Operative and patient care techniques for posterior mini-incision total hip arthroplasty. *Clin Orthop Relat Res* 2005;441:104-114.

22. Goldstein W, Branson J, Berland K, Gordon A: Minimal-incision total hip arthroplasty. *J Bone Joint Surg Am* 2003;85:33-38.

23. Wright J, Crockett H, Delgado S, Lyman S, Madsen M, Sculco T: Mini-incision for total hip arthroplasty: A prospective, controlled investigation with 5 year follow-up evaluation. *J Arthroplasty* 2004;19:538-545.

24. Chimento G, Pavone V, Sharrock N, Kahn B, Cahill J, Sculco T: Minimally invasive total hip arthroplasty: A prospective randomized study. *J Arthroplasty* 2005;20:139-144.

25. Ogonda L, Wilson R, Archbold P, et al: A minimal-incision technique in total hip arthroplasty does not improve early postoperative outcomes: A prospective, randomized, controlled trial. *J Bone Joint Surg Am* 2005;87:701-710.

26. Swanson T: Early results of 1000 consecutive, posterior, single-incision minimally invasive surgery total hip arthroplasties. *J Arthroplasty* 2005;20(Suppl 3):26-32.

27. Woolson ST, Mow C, Syquia J, Lannin J, Schurman D: Comparison of primary total hip replacements performed with standard incision or a mini-incision. *J Bone Joint Surg Am* 2004;86:1353-1358.

28. Berger R, Jacobs J, Meneghini M, Della Valle C, Paprosky W, Rosenberg A: Rapid rehabilitation and recovery with minimally invasive total hip arthroplasty. *Clin Orthop Relat Res* 2004;429:239-247.

29. Mardones R, Pagnano M, Nemanich J, Trousdale R: Muscle damage after total hip arthroplasty done with the two-incision and mini-posterior techniques. *Clin Orthop Relat Res* 2005;441:63-67.

30. Wixson RL, MacDonald MA: Total hip arthroplasty through a minimal posterior approach using imageless computer-assisted hip navigation. *J Arthroplasty* 2005;20(Suppl 3):51-56.

# CHAPTER 6

# RAPID RECOVERY FOLLOWING LIMITED INCISION TOTAL HIP ARTHROPLASTY

KEITH R. BEREND, MD
ADOLPH V. LOMBARDI, JR, MD, FACS

Since the original descriptions of Sir John Charnley,[1] the primary goals of total hip arthroplasty (THA) have remained relatively unchanged. Those goals include pain relief, restoration of function, and improvement in quality of life. In recent years, surgeons have sought to achieve these goals with reduced hospital stays and quicker recovery times. Measurement of success and failure in THA has been constantly evaluated with a primary focus on relief of pain.[2] Whereas relief of pain is a critical component for a successful outcome, excellent and speedy functional recovery is also important. Rapid recovery and rehabilitation focuses on measures of recovery such as hospital length of stay, the length of time until assistive devices can be discontinued, and the use of postoperative rehabilitation services.

The burgeoning interest in limited incision techniques for THA has created a push to shorten the timeline of recovery and elevated the level of functional recovery that the patient and surgeon expect from THA. Less damage to soft tissues that allows for a faster functional recovery is the keystone to a program of limited incision surgery. It is, however, the constantly changing and evolving rehabilitation and pain management protocols that have provided the foundation of this technical revolution. Less invasive surgery alone cannot provide rapid recovery from THA. Instead, multimodal pain management and a holistic approach to the care of the patient and family are responsible for much of the progress seen in THA rehabilitation.[3]

Many factors related to the implant, surgeon, hospital, and patient have been identified as important variables in postoperative patient recovery and the subsequent success of THA. Patient factors include: age, race, gender, education, social support, medical comorbidities, and primary hip pathology. Surgeon factors include surgical experience, surgical volume, surgical approach, and technical completion of the procedure.

Hospital variables include volume, rehabilitation protocols, clinical care pathways, and anesthetic technique.[4] No single variable is entirely responsible for improvement; all work in synergy to provide a rapid functional recovery and successful long-term arthroplasty construct. In this chapter we will review the recent advancements in rehabilitation protocols, multimodal pain management, and adjunct materials and methods for rapid recovery following THA.

## BACKGROUND

Even in early publications on outcomes in THA, investigators identified physical therapy as an important factor in the recovery following THA.[5,6] Charnley[1] originally reported immobilization for 3 weeks in plaster splints and a hospital length of stay of 8 weeks. From this starting point, rapid recovery techniques and limited incision surgery have pushed the limits of THA to overnight hospital stays and even outpatient surgery status.[7] We have previously published a review of principles of rapid recovery, including early outcomes of their implementation.[3] This program involves preoperative patient and family education, perioperative nutrition and smoking cessation, preemptive and multimodal analgesia, perioperative rehabilitation, and clinical care pathways in combination with less invasive surgical techniques. Credit and recognition is due to Marshall Steele, MD,[8,9] an innovator and pioneer in the area of improving outcomes and patient satisfaction, particularly in the perioperative period. Much of our current protocols and perioperative programs has been influenced by Dr. Steele's work in this swiftly expanding area of healthcare.

## PREOPERATIVE EDUCATION AND REHABILITATION

Patient preoperative education has been the subject of recent efforts in THA surgery. By educating the patient and family on the technical aspects of the procedure, undue anxiety and fears are reduced. Lee and Gin[10] reported a reduction in patient anxiety after a multidisciplinary healthcare team conducted a small group program. Information leaflets describing various anesthetic techniques also were used but were not found to be as useful as the small group sessions.

The office environment is an ideal place to begin the culture of healing and education. Office flip charts that contain simple illustrations of arthritic conditions and THA prostheses are available in each examination room. Following an initial evaluation by a qualified physician extender such as a nurse practitioner or physician assistant, the patient and family are encouraged to browse the flip charts in anticipation of questions that may arise during the physician encounter (**Figure 1**). We use educational workbooks that are given to the patient and family when surgery is scheduled (**Figure 2**). These books contain detailed information covering everything from directions to the hospital, what to expect before, during, and after the surgery, and postoperative rehabilitation exercises. Specific exercises and postoperative restrictions are tailored to the patient depending on medical comorbidities such as dementia and implant type (**Figure 3**). For example, in patients who receive a large diameter metal-on-metal articulation, postoperative dislocation precautions are lessened and the patient is allowed a quicker return to normal activities.

Preoperative education also includes an individually tailored preoperative physical therapy evaluation that has been previously demonstrated to reduce hospital length of stay[11] (**Figure 4**). Further reductions in length of stay, improved outcomes, and better patient satisfaction are also gained by the use of preadmission social services screening. By identifying and addressing, preoperatively, the needs of the individual patient and family, coordination of care and discharge plans can be set up ahead of time, allowing for an earlier discharge to home or an extended care facility. Many wasted hospital days are spent coordinating discharge planning, when these easily could be saved with preadmission planning.[12] Preoperative education not only effectively reduces the hospital stay but has also been correlated with a reduction in pain medication usage by patients with the most anxiety and denial in a study by Daltroy and associates.[13] They report that these types of patients may be difficult to identify, and thus all patients should undergo extensive preoperative education and rehabilitation to provide the most significant response. Overall, preoperative education and rehabilitation training have been shown to reduce hospital length of stay and improve patient and family satisfaction.[14]

Preoperative education also includes a discussion with the patient and family regarding smoking cessation and nutritional status. Multiple studies have linked postop-

FIGURE 1

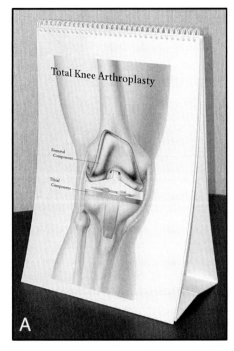
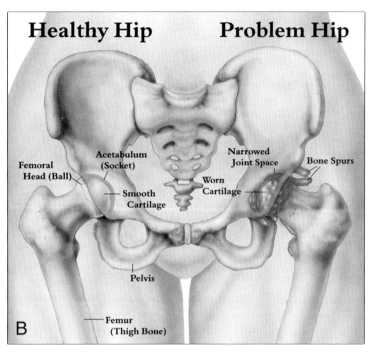

A, Flip charts, developed by our in-house staff artist, illustrating arthritic conditions and arthroplasty of the hip and knee are available in each patient examination room. These charts provide information about the arthritic condition and the surgical intervention, and the patient is encouraged to view these while waiting. B, Simple to understand medical illustrations by our staff artist outlining arthritis and total hip arthroplasty procedures are contained within the examination room flip chart. (Reproduced with permission of Joint Implant Surgeons, Inc.)

erative medical and orthopaedic complications to smoking.[15-17] Smoking is, in fact, considered the single most significant risk factor for complications following elective THA.[15] Smoking cessation education and intervention can be effective in reducing the perioperative complication rate, however, and all surgeons should screen patients and provide the appropriate educational materials and opportunities for their patients to quit.[16]

The preoperative nutritional status also is of particular importance because malnutrition is linked to medical and surgical complications.[18,19] Among the routine medical screening laboratory tests obtained before surgery, a simple battery of serum parameters can be obtained to identify the patient at risk for complications secondary to poor nutrition. These tests include serum albumin, serum transferrin, and total lymphocyte count.[18-20] A low serum albumin, in particular, has been associated with increased length of stay and increased cost of care. Serum zinc levels have been linked to delayed wound healing in hip hemiarthroplasty for fracture, and may well represent another target for preoperative screening in elective THA.[21] Patients diagnosed with malnutrition preoperatively can be delayed and referred to a nutritionist for education and counseling.

Obesity is a rising epidemic in the United States. Morbid obesity makes THA technically more challenging, and some believe that obesity may dissuade surgeons from offering THA in otherwise appropriate candidates.[22] Any discussion of minimally invasive or mini-incision THA routinely excludes the morbidly obese patient. In these patients, who may not be candidates for less invasive THA, a rapid rehabilitation program may still be effective. The results in terms of improvement in quality of life following THA in obese patients are not significantly different than those in patients of more normal weight.[23] Obesity, however, has been linked to risk of wound infection, deep venous thrombosis, and pulmonary embolism.[24-26] Delay in rehabilitation,

## FIGURE 2

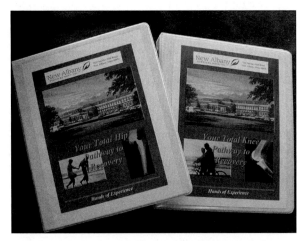

Guidebooks, developed by our staff in collaboration with our hospital and physical therapy professionals, are specifically designed for total hip and total knee arthroplasty and are given to the patient at the time that the surgical procedure is scheduled. These books contain vital information regarding the hospital, the surgical intervention, how to prepare for surgery, details about discharge disposition, exercises, and expectations. (Reproduced with permission of Joint Implant Surgeons, Inc.)

## FIGURE 3

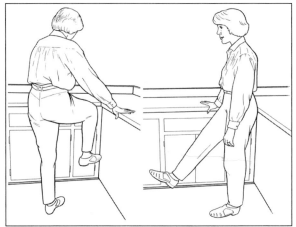

The guidebooks contain illustrations and descriptions of specific exercises that the patient is to practice before surgery. Exercises can be highlighted or excluded based on patient and implant factors. (Reproduced with permission of Joint Implant Surgeons, Inc.)

increased requirements for aid and assistance, and an overall slower recovery are also noted in obese lower extremity patients in our practice. Therefore, it is the role of the orthopedic surgeon to have a candid discussion regarding obesity. We currently offer referral to a weight loss surgery center for consideration of bariatric surgery to our obese patients. Previous work has shown that bariatric surgery prior to arthroplasty is effective in allowing for massive weight loss and enabling a full and rapid functional recovery in most patients who elect to undergo this type of procedure before elective THA.[27]

Lastly, patient and family education involves setting realistic expectations for the recovery process in terms of both short- and long-term outcomes. This includes upfront discussions about hospital length of stay. If patients and family are informed of an early discharge and are invested in this concept, patient satisfaction is maintained while efficiency is increased. A candid discussion regarding short- and long-term activity restrictions needs to take place preoperatively. The boon of less invasive surgery can lead patients to have unrealistic expectations of the recovery and the long-term outcomes. Regardless of the surgical technique and surgical

approach, THA is a serious undertaking and the patient and family need to realize this preoperatively.

## CLINICAL CARE PATHWAYS AND MAPS

The concept of standardized care for a particular single procedure is an attractive way to increase efficiency. Regardless of implant selection, patient characteristics, and surgical approach, the surgical intervention of THA is basically the same in most patients. For most cases, patients respond and recover within one standard deviation of each other. For that reason, most patients can be treated in a relatively standardized fashion. One of the most critical aspects of the perioperative experience is allowing the patient and family to feel special and individualized while still maintaining a standardized plan for their recovery. The best way to accomplish this feat is to allow the physician and physician extenders to care directly for the individual patient and spend time listening to concerns and feelings while having the care team follow a preordained plan of care.

Another important aspect of individualized care is preemptively educating the patient and family as to the plan of postoperative care. To avoid potential frustration or a feeling that the patient requires a longer hospital

FIGURE 4

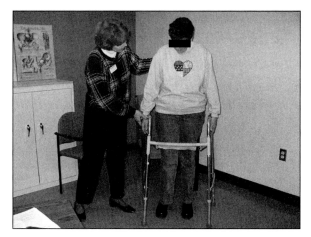

All patients are evaluated and examined by a physical therapist with an emphasis on postoperative exercises. Severe preoperative limp, limb-length inequality, and motor weakness is evaluated and preemptively addressed. Instruction on the proper use of assistive devices is provided. (Reproduced with permission of Joint Implant Surgeons, Inc.)

stay, the patient and family should be familiarized with the planned hospital stay, discharge disposition, and follow-up plans well in advance. The entire care team should then reinforce the same concepts throughout the surgical experience.

Fisher and associates[28] investigated a specialized patient management system for the hospital care of the lower extremity arthroplasty patient. They reported a significant reduction in length of stay and hospital charges in all procedural categories, including primary and revision hip and knee arthroplasty. Using a preestablished clinical pathway for standardized care of the arthroplasty patient, we have also observed a reduction in average acute length of stay without increasing utilization of post-discharge facilities, and with no increase in complications. Data such as this prove that rapid recovery and earlier discharge for the acute care setting does not endanger the patient or shift the burden of care to the rehabilitation setting. With a goal of early hospital discharge (or overnight stay THA surgery), it should be noted that not all patients will be discharged directly to home within 24 hours of surgery. We have observed a rule of thirds in our recovery program. Approximately one third of patients are safely discharged to home within 24 hours of surgery, the next one third of patients

require a hospital stay of 2 days to achieve the goals for safe discharge, and the final one third require a 3-day hospital stay with or without discharge to a skilled facility or rehabilitation center. It is relatively easy to classify patients into these categories preoperatively. Younger appearing patients with fewer medical comorbidities, strong social support, and moderate preoperative functional loss can be targeted for discharge within 24 hours. Elderly, frail patients who may live alone and possess little social and family support will most likely require an extended rehabilitation stay and can be slated for a 3-day hospital stay prior to admission. Forrest and associates[29] categorized patients as likely to require a rehabilitation facility stay if they are older, live alone, and have an American Society of Anesthesiologists (ASA) score of 3 or 4. This concept of a standardized clinical care pathway with two or more patient categories was described by Wang and associates.[30] They noted that there was a bimodal distribution of when patients achieved the recovery of functional independence. Simple screening using ASA guidelines, type of social situation, and patient preoperative functional status can identify those patients who will be able to go home within 24 hours and those that will require a rehabilitation stay.

Over the past decade, these so-called care maps have become the standard of care in most orthopaedic centers. By virtue of the homogeneous nature of the THA procedure itself, THA is the ideal platform for standardization of hospital care. Multiple studies have proven that length of stay can be reduced with an associated significant cost savings to patient, insurance carrier, and hospital system without compromising the results or increasing complications. Healy and associates[31] demonstrated a reduction in cost and length of stay with the use of clinical pathways without shifting the burden of care to rehabilitation centers. In the largest review of the subject, Kim and associates[32] performed a meta-analysis to determine the utility of care maps and clinical pathways in THA and TKA procedures. They concluded that based on a review of the published information, clinical pathways effectively reduce cost and length of stay with no negative compromise in outcomes. One critical aspect of a uniform hospital-wide clinical pathway for the care of the arthroplasty patient is enrolling the support of all surgeons and caregivers involved. Establishing a clinical pathway is a constantly evolving process that requires constant review and restructuring and the participation and input from all the caregivers involved.

## PREEMPTIVE ANALGESIA

Following patient and family education, the next most important factor in providing an atmosphere of healing is adequate reduction and control of pain. Even the least invasive THA requires cutting bone and insertion of a prosthesis into the host bone; therefore, some pain is expected. Preemptively attacking pain is crucial to allowing a quick recovery. Beginning preoperatively, the noxious stimuli of surgery must be blocked. This is accomplished by a multimodal approach. Preoperative administration of anti-inflammatory medications combined with a multimodal anesthetic protocol provides the most efficient means of controlling postoperative pain. We have investigated this phenomenon in multiple studies.[33-35] Using a formal perioperative pain management protocol, our patients are out of bed participating in physical therapy within hours of the surgical intervention.[35,36] This perioperative pain management protocol involves the use of preoperative COX-2 nonsteroidal anti-inflammatory medications. The use of COX-2 preoperatively and in the immediate postoperative period reduces postoperative narcotic usage, decreases the incidence of nausea, and prevents confusion.[34,37] We prescribe celecoxib 200 mg to be taken the day before surgery and continued for 2 weeks postoperatively. Additionally, oxycodone, a long-acting slow-release narcotic, is administered (20 mg for patients younger than age 70 and 10 mg for patients older than age 70 years) every 12 hours beginning 2 hours after arrival to the hospital floor. Oral narcotics are used as needed throughout the hospital period and on discharge. While some investigators have recommended preoperative administration of narcotics, we avoid doing so because of our use of intrathecal narcotics.

For surgical analgesia, we prefer a single shot spinal anesthetic with morphine (200 to 300 mcg) and bupivacaine (7.5 to 12.5 mg). This combination provides adequate surgical anesthesia and postoperative pain control for several hours. This allows the oral long-acting narcotic to build up to adequate serum levels without the need for intravenous medications. Others have advocated the use of a "3-in-1" block for THA postoperative analgesia. This block involves a proximal sciatic blockade to block the posterior thigh and leg, excluding saphenous distribution combined with a psoas compartment blockade to block the lumbar plexus.[38-40] This is an effective method when combined with oral narcotics, local wound blockade, and oral COX-2 medications.

At the local wound site, a soft-tissue injection containing 60 mL of 0.5% ropivacaine with 0.5 mg epinephrine and 30 mg of ketorolac (contraindicated in patients with renal insufficiency, history of allergy to nonsteroidal anti-inflammatory drugs, or a creatinine level higher than 1.5) is used. These injection cocktails appear safe and effective for not only improving pain and swelling but also providing a level of hemostasis. The injection is given directly into the capsule, muscles, fascial planes, and subcutaneously. Strong support for this type of local wound block is seen in the total knee arthroplasty (TKA) literature.[41,42] Despite the use of regional blockade, soft-tissue injections serve an important role in multimodal analgesia by targeting the local pain receptors and reducing inflammatory response. The combined effect of the ropivacaine and ketorolac has been reported to last up to 24 hours.

One important factor in the use of intrathecal narcotics is preemptively addressing the resulting nausea. Preoperatively, all patients are given an intravenous dose of steroid, 4 mg dexamethasone, and an antiemetic, 4 mg ondansetron. A single sea-sickness patch containing transdermal scopolamine, is also placed prior to induction of the spinal anesthetic and removed on postoperative day one. This protocol effectively eliminates most of the nausea caused by the use of a spinal narcotic. Postoperatively, ondansetron is used for an antiemetic.

These multimodal pathways for analgesia were recently reviewed by Horlocker and associates.[39] They concluded that a multimodal pathway encompassing preemptive treatment with oral narcotics and COX-2 inhibitors combined with a peripheral nerve block is the most effective program for pain control following TKA and THA. We would emphasize that peripheral nerve blocks can be technically challenging and time consuming. We have had a great deal of success with a similar program of preemptive analgesia combined with intraoperative soft-tissue local wound block, spinal local anesthetic, and narcotic anesthesia. Preoperative oral narcotics are not given because intrathecal narcotics are administered. Control of iatrogenic side effects such as

## FIGURE 5

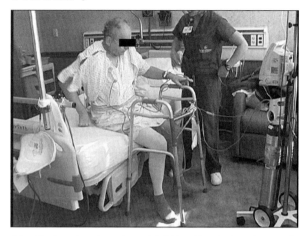

All patients undergoing primary total hip arthroplasty undergo early postoperative therapy. This consists of ambulation within hours of arrival to the inpatient care unit. Mobility and independence are encouraged when safe. Allowing patients to ambulate in the early postoperative period, when pain is controlled by the long-acting spinal anesthetic, provides positive reinforcement and may reduce the incidence of thromboembolic disease. (Reproduced with permission of Joint Implant Surgeons, Inc.)

nausea is critical, and consultation with the local anesthesia team is essential in providing a uniform yet effective program.

## POSTOPERATIVE THERAPY

In the culture of healing that is established by "prehabilitation," education, and preemptive analgesia, postoperative therapy becomes the next step following limited incision THA. We use an aggressive program emphasizing mobility and independence. All patients undergoing primary THA at our institution ambulate within hours of arrival to the unit on the day of surgery (**Figure 5**). We allow immediate weight bearing as tolerated with the use of an assistive device such as a walker or cane. Immediate weight bearing and mobility appears to be safe as we have encouraged this for all patients despite our use of cementless fixation.[43,44] This is an especially crucial timeframe for patient ambulation. Being able to walk without pain in the early postoperative period provides a mental and emotional stimulation to the patient and family. Early mobilization is also an effective adjunct for the prevention of thromboembolic disease.[45]

On the morning following surgery, the indwelling catheter is discontinued and further ambulation is undertaken. Patients receive therapy twice a day prior to discharge. The patients are then taken to the hospital stairwell where they are assisted with climbing and descending stairs. Stair climbing and the ability to independently transfer into and out of a bed and chair are the requisites for discharge to home. We do not routinely use outpatient or home health therapy following THA. For this reason, preoperative education and rehabilitation are essential.

The patient guidebooks contain an outline and timeline for activity and exercise. The patients are encouraged to discontinue the use of assistive devices when pain has subsided and the limp has returned to preoperative severity. Most patients are either using a cane for long distances or no assistive device by the 6-week follow-up examination. During routine 6-week follow-up, the patient is evaluated for residual limp or abductor weakness. If these are present, the patients are referred to our therapist for a one-time evaluation and education visit. Return to work status is individualized on a per-patient basis depending on occupation and recreational activities.

It cannot be overemphasized that the preoperative education and instruction on postoperative activities and exercise are critical to rapid recovery. Patients who have undergone intensive preoperative counseling and evaluation by a physical therapist have been shown to recover function significantly faster than those who received in-hospital therapy alone.[46] We constantly encourage patients to practice and perform the exercises that are contained within the guidebook during the time leading up to the surgical intervention. Instructions that further encourage performance of the prescribed exercises are given to the patient going home. Patients are also instructed to ambulate as tolerated daily following discharge.

## RESULTS AND CONCLUSIONS

The isolated benefits of performing limited incision THA procedure have been debated. There are conflicting reports touting quicker recovery and less pain and others reporting no benefit from smaller incision techniques.[47-52] We have previously reported on the positive effects of a rapid recovery program in traditional open

FIGURE 6

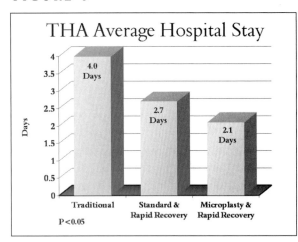

To isolate the effect of a less invasive approach, three groups were retrospectively examined. The traditional group serves as a historic control with an average length of stay (LOS) of 4.0 days. The addition of a holistic perioperative program, with a standard anterolateral approach (standard and rapid recovery) demonstrated a reduction in length of stay to 2.7 days.[3] A further significant reduction in average LOS of 0.6 days was observed with the addition of the Microplasty (Biomet, Inc, Warsaw, IN) anterolateral approach to the rapid recovery program (Microplasty and rapid recovery; $P < 0.05$). (Reproduced with permission of Joint Implant Surgeons, Inc.)

THA techniques with a reduction in length of stay and hospital readmission rates.[3] Further evaluation has shown that the addition of a less invasive technique can further safely reduce hospital length of stay. Our previous report examined a group of traditional open THAs prior to implementation of the rapid recovery program as a control group (traditional).[5] The average length of stay in this group was 4.0 days. The second group consisted of a traditional open incision and the aforementioned rapid recovery program (standard and rapid recovery). The average length of stay was 2.7 days. When a less invasive Microplasty (Biomet, Inc, Warsaw, IN) anterolateral approach was added to the holistic program, a significant further reduction in length of stay of 0.6 days ($P < 0.5$) was observed (Microplasty and rapid recovery) with an average stay of 2.1 days. These results are illustrated in **Figure 6**. It should be noted that the most significant reduction was achieved by the addition of a holistic recovery program with a more modest reduction seen with less invasive surgery.

Regardless of a surgeon's personal perspective or level of comfort with the various less invasive techniques, it is certain that our continual evaluation and improvement of the pre- and postoperative care of the THA patient has had a substantial positive impact on outcomes. The combination of less invasive techniques and newer perioperative protocols for patient care has consistently shown improved early results with less pain, quicker recovery, and improved patient satisfaction.[5,48,53] It is the care of the patient, the patient's family, and the patient's pain that provide better early outcomes. When combined with less invasive techniques, a rapid recovery program provides clear benefits to both the patient and the caregivers. The THA surgeon's role as physician and the care of the entire patient may well be more important than the surgical technique.

## References

1. Charnley J: Arthroplasty of the hip: A new operation. *Lancet* 1961;1:1129-1132.

2. Harris WH: Traumatic arthritis of the hip after dislocation and acetabular fractures: Treatment by mold arthroplasty. *J Bone Joint Surg Am* 1969;51:737-755.

3. Berend KR, Lombard AV Jr, Mallory TH: Rapid recovery protocol for peri-operative care of total hip and total knee arthroplasty patients. *Surg Technol Int* 2004;14:239-247.

4. Lang MH, Katz JN, Phillips C, et al: The total hip arthroplasty outcome evaluation form of the American Academy of Orthopaedic Surgeons: Results of a nominal group process. *J Bone Joint Surg Am* 1991;73:639-646.

5. Richardson RW: Physical therapy management of patients undergoing total hip replacement. *Phys Ther* 1975;55:984-989.

6. Opitz JL: Total joint arthroplasty: Principles and guidelines for postoperative physiatric management. *Mayo Clin Proc* 1979;54:602-612.

7. Ilfeld BM, Gearen PF, Enneking FK, et al: Total hip arthroplasty as an overnight-stay procedure using an ambulatory continuous psoas compartment nerve block: A prospective feasibility study. *Reg Anesth Pain Med* 2006;31:113-118.

8. Steele MK III, McLean MB, Gaunt R, Browning WA: The Joint Ventures program: Improving outcomes and satisfaction in joint surgery patients. *J Clin Outcomes Manage* 2000;7(7):28-30.

9.  Steele MK: Surgeons/hospitals: It's time to sharpen your saw. *Orthop Product News* 2005;July/August:33-34.

10. Lee A, Gin T: Educating patients about anesthesia: Effects of various modes on patients' knowledge, anxiety, and satisfaction. *Curr Opin Anaesthesiol* 2005;18:205-208.

11. Crowe J, Henderson J: Pre-arthroplasty rehabilitation is effective in reducing hospital stay. *Can J Occup Ther* 2003;70:88-96.

12. Liebergall M, Soskoline V, Mattan Y, et al: Preadmission screening of patients scheduled for hip and knee replacement: Impact on length of stay. *Clin Perform Qual Health Care* 1999;7:17-22.

13. Daltroy LH, Morlino CI, Eaton HM, et al: Preoperative education for total hip and knee replacement patients. *Arthritis Care Res* 1998;11:469-478.

14. McGregor AH, Rylands H, Owen A, Dore CJ, Hughes SP: Does preoperative hip rehabilitation advice improve recovery and patient satisfaction? *J Arthroplasty* 2004;19(4):464-468.

15. Moller AM, Pedersen T, Villebro N, et al: Effect of smoking on early complications after elective orthopedic surgery. *J Bone Joint Surg Br* 2003;85:178-181.

16. Moller AM, Villebro N, Pedersen T, Tonnesen H: Effect of preoperative smoking intervention on postoperative complications: A randomized clinical trial. *Lancet* 2002;359:114-117.

17. Lavernia CJ, Sierra RJ, Gomez-Martin O: Smoking and joint replacement: Resource consumption and short term outcome. *Clin Orthop Relat Res* 1999;367:172-180.

18. Lavernia CJ, Sierra RJ, Baerga L: Nutritional parameters and short term outcome in arthroplasty. *J Am Col Nutr* 1999;18:274-278.

19. Gherini S, Vaughn BK, Lombardi AV Jr, Mallory TH: Delayed wound healing and nutritional deficiencies after total hip arthroplasty. *Clin Orthop Relat Res* 1993;293:188-195.

20. Del Savio GC, Zelicof SB, Wexler LM, et al: Preoperative nutritional status and outcome of elective total hip replacement. *Clin Orthop Relat Res* 1996;326:153-161.

21. Zorrilla P, Salido JA, Lopez-Alonso A, Silva A: Serum zinc as a prognostic tool for wound healing in hip hemiarthroplasty. *Clin Orthop Relat Res* 2004;420:304-308.

22. Naik G: Surgeons' weighty dilemma; wary of the risk, work, some doctors won't replace knees, hips of obese patients. *Wall St J* (East Ed) 2006;Feb 28:B1, B8.

23. Chan CL, Villar RN: Obesity and quality of life after primary hip arthroplasty. *J Bone Joint Surg Br* 1996;78:78-81.

24. Namba RS, Paxton L, Fithian DC, Stone ML: Obesity and perioperative morbidity in total hip and knee arthroplasty patients. *J Arthroplasty* 2005;20(7 Suppl 3):46-50.

25. Bagaria V, Modi N, Panghate A, Vaidya S: Incidence and risk factors for development of venous thromboembolism in Indian patients undergoing major orthopaedic surgery: Results of a prospective study. *Postgrad Med J* 2006;82:136-139.

26. Mantilla CB, Horlocker TT, Schroeder DR, et al: Risk factors for clinically relevant pulmonary embolism and deep venous thrombosis in patients undergoing primary hip or knee arthroplasty. *Anesthesiology* 2003;99:552-560.

27. Parvizi J, Trousdale RT, Sarr MG: Total joint arthroplasty in patients surgically treated for morbid obesity. *J Arthroplasty* 2000;15:1003-1008.

28. Fisher DA, Trimble S, Clapp B, Dorsett K: Effect of a patient management system on outcomes of total hip and knee arthroplasty. *Clin Orthop Relat Res* 1997;345:155-160.

29. Forrest GP, Roque JM, Dawodu ST: Decreasing length of stay after total joint arthroplasty: Effect on referrals to rehabilitation units. *Arch Phys Med Rehabil* 1999;80:192-194.

30. Wang A, Hall S, Gilbey H, Ackland T: Patient variability and the design of clinical pathways after primary total hip replacement surgery. *J Qual Clin Pract* 1997;17:123-129.

31. Healy WL, Ayers ME, Iorio R, et al: Impact of a clinical pathway and implant standardization on total hip arthroplasty: A clinical and economic study of short-term patient outcomes. *J Arthroplasty* 1998;13:266-276.

32. Kim S, Losina E, Solomon DH, Wright J, Katz JN: Effectiveness of clinical pathways for total knee and total hip arthroplasty: Literature review. *J Arthroplasty* 2003;18:69-74.

33. Mallory TH, Lombardi AV Jr, Fada RA, et al: Anesthesia options: Choices and caveats. *Orthopedics* 2000;23:919-920.

34. Mallory TH, Lombardi AV Jr, Fada RA, et al: Pain management for total joint arthroplasty: Preemptive analgesia. *J Arthroplasty* 2002;17:129-133.

35. Dodds KL, Adams JB, Russell JH, et al: Pain management for the total knee arthroplasty patient: A multimodal management model featuring soft-tissue and intra-articular injection. NAON 23rd Annual Congress Proceedings: Orlando, FL, 2003.

36. Lombardi AV Jr, Berend KR, Mallory TH, Dodds KL, Adams JB: Soft-tissue and intra-articular bupivacaine, epinephrine and narcotic injection in knee arthroplasty. *Clin Orthop Relat Res* 2004;248:125-130.

37. Buvanendran A, Kroin JS, Turman KJ, et al: The effect of peri-operative administration of a selective cyclooxygenase-2 inhibitor on pain management and function after total knee replacement: A randomized controlled trial. *JAMA* 2003;290:2411-2418.

38. Singelyn FJ, Gouverneur JM: Postoperative analgesia after total hip arthroplasty: IV PCA with morphine, patient-controlled epidural analgesia, or continuous "3-in-1" block? A prospective evaluation by our acute pain service in more than 1300 patients. *J Clin Anesth* 1999;11:550-554.

39. Horlocker TT, Kopp SL, Pagnano MW, Hebl JR: Analgesia for total hip and knee arthroplasty: A multimodal pathway featuring peripheral nerve block. *J Am Acad Orthop Surg* 2006;14:126-135.

40. Capdevila X, Macaire P, Dadure C, et al: Continuous psoas compartment block for postoperative analgesia after total hip arthroplasty: New landmarks, technical guidelines, and clinical evaluation. *Anesth Analg* 2004;98:1606-1613.

41. Vendittoli PA, Makinen P, Drolet P, et al: A multimodal analgesia protocol for total knee arthroplasty: A randomized, controlled study. *J Bone Joint Surg Am* 2006;88:273-281.

42. Lombardi AV Jr, Berend KR, Mallory TH, et al: Soft tissue and intra-articular injection of bupivacaine, epinephrine, and morphine has a beneficial effect after total knee arthroplasty. *Clin Orthop Relat Res* 2004;428:125-130.

43. Berend KR, Lombardi AV Jr, Mallory TH, et al: Cerclage wires or cables for the management of intraoperative fracture associated with a cementless, tapered femoral prosthesis: Results at 2 to 16 years. *J Arthroplasty* 2004;19:17-21.

44. Boden H, Adolphson P: No adverse effects of early weight bearing after uncemented total hip arthroplasty: A randomized study of 20 patients. *Acta Orthop Scand* 2004;75:21-29.

45. Berend KR, Lombardi AV Jr: Multimodal venous thromboembolic disease prevention for patients undergoing primary or revision total joint arthroplasty: The role of aspirin. *Am J Orthop* 2006;35:24-29.

46. Gilbey HJ, Ackland TR, Wang AW, et al: Exercise improves early functional recovery after total hip arthroplasty. *Clin Orthop Relat Res* 2003;408:193-200.

47. Jerosch J, Thaising C, Fadel ME: Antero-lateral minimal invasive (ALMI) approach for total hip arthroplasty technique and early results. *Arch Orthop Trauma Surg* 2006;126:164-173.

48. Inaba Y, Dorr LD, Wan Z, et al: Operative and patient care techniques for posterior mini-incision total hip arthroplasty. *Clin Orthop Relat Res* 2005;441:104-114.

49. O'Brien DA, Rorabeck CH: The mini-incision direct lateral approach in primary total hip arthroplasty. *Clin Orthop Relat Res* 2005;441:99-103.

50. Pagnano MW, Leone J, Lewallen DG, Hanssen AD: Two-incision THA had modest outcomes and some substantial complications. *Clin Orthop Relat Res* 2005;441:86-90.

51. Suzuki K, Kawachi S, Sakai H, et al: Mini-incision total hip arthroplasty: A quantitative assessment of laboratory data and clinical outcomes. *J Orthop Sci* 2004;9:571-575.

52. Swanson TV: Early results of 1000 consecutive, posterior, single-incision minimally invasive surgery total hip arthroplasties. *J Arthroplasty* 2005;20:26-32.

53. Peck CN, Foster A, McLauchlan GJ: Reducing incision length or intensifying rehabilitation: What makes the difference to length of stay in total hip replacement in a UK setting? *Int Orthop* 2006;30:395-398.

# INDEX

## T

*American Academy of Orthopaedic Surgeons*